LACAN AND THE FORMULAE OF SEXUATION

Lacan and the Formulae of Sexuation provides the first critical reading of Lacan's formulae of sexuation, examining both their logical consistency and clinical consequences. Are there two different entities named Man and Woman, separated by the gulf of sexual difference? Or is it better to conceive of this difference as something purely relative, each human being situated on a sort of continuum from more or less 'man' to more or less 'woman'?

Sigmund Freud established the strange way through which sexuality determines being human: his concept of drive was no longer the heteronormative sexual instinct used by the psychiatrists of his time. With his provocative formula according to which 'there is no sexual relationship', Lacan has reinforced this perspective, combining logic and sexuality through the invention of a new operator, the concept 'not-all', which points to a form of incompleteness at stake in his 'formulae of sexuation'. This book examines how these formulae have been constructed, and how we should read them in connection with, on one hand, their own logical consistency (a logical square different from Aristotelian tradition) and, on the other hand, a 'part object' in a very different sense to Melanie Klein's. The book also investigates the underlying logic of clinical vignettes, so much in favour in psychoanalytical literature today.

The book represents essential reading for Lacanian psychoanalysts, as well as researchers at the cross-section of psychoanalysis, philosophy, and gender studies.

Guy Le Gaufey was a member of the Ecole Freudienne de Paris and co-founded the Lacanian journal *Littoral* and the *École lacanienne de psychanalyse*. He has written and published widely in French, English, and Spanish and has also translated books from English to French, including the work of Philip Larkin (see www.legaufey.fr).

LACAN AND THE FORMULAE OF SEXUATION

Exploring Logical Consistency and Clinical Consequences

Guy Le Gaufey

TRANSLATED BY CORMAC GALLAGHER

Routledge
Taylor & Francis Group
LONDON AND NEW YORK

First published in English 2020
by Routledge
2 Park Square, Milton Park, Abingdon, Oxon OX14 4RN

and by Routledge
52 Vanderbilt Avenue, New York, NY 10017

Routledge is an imprint of the Taylor & Francis Group, an informa business

Original title: Le Pas tout de Lacan

Published by arrangement with Agence litteraire Astier-Pécher

British Library Cataloguing-in-Publication Data
A catalogue record for this book is available from the British Library

Library of Congress Cataloging-in-Publication Data
Names: Le Gaufey, Guy, author.
Title: Lacan and the formulae of sexuation : exploring logical consistency and clinical consequences / Guy Le Gaufey ; translated by Cormac Gallagher.
Other titles: Pastout de Lacan, consistance logique, conséquences cliniques. English
Description: 1 Edition. | New York : Routledge, 2020. | Includes bibliographical references and index.
Identifiers: LCCN 2019038843 | ISBN 9780367420468 (hardback) | ISBN 9780367420376 (paperback) | ISBN 9780367821456 (ebook)
Subjects: LCSH: Lacan, Jacques, 1901–1981. | Psychoanalysis—France—History—20th century.
Classification: LCC BF109.L28 L4413 2020 | DDC 150.19/5092—dc23
LC record available at https://lccn.loc.gov/2019038843

ISBN: 978-0-367-42046-8 (hbk)
ISBN: 978-0-367-42037-6 (pbk)
ISBN: 978-0-367-82145-6 (ebk)

Typeset in Bembo
by Apex CoVantage, LLC

CONTENTS

PROLOGUE

Scarcely has one been convinced that the attraction described as sexual is not reduced to the interplay of pheromones but is going to draw considerable resources from the symbolic material that is so pregnant in this species that one sees there opening up a curious questioning: If there are two sexes, which attract one another, which is the one and which is the other? 'It's all the same!' our contemporaries will say; each is the other of the other – therefore each is one. I propose in what follows not to go so quickly and to take the time required to go from one to two imposing that this latter ought to be the other of the first. Here already logical concern shows the tip of its nose. We have a presentiment that the otherness at the heart of a couple is not the one that is established in the heart of a plurality and that the difference which separates one from the other is perhaps not proper to either the one nor the other. In any case, things become complicated in the measure that the basic logical instruments – the same, the other, difference, property, the identical – are from the very start required to articulate anything whatsoever about the sexes *in the discursive order.* Could it be that the noble philosophical clothing of these instruments is, in fact, completely impregnated by the hollow quarrel of the sexes and that certain logical pillars (and some foundations of this social order) have been constructed to rule over a sexual confusion considered to be fatal? Very early on, people began to think, including logically, *against* the sexual thing?

This is a hypothesis that Jacques Lacan seems to have made. He has scarcely attempted to organise the two sexes when we see him appealing to the arsenal of traditional logic of universal affirmative and negative propositions, accompanied by their respective particulars. After a salvo that was isolated for a long time (at the beginning of 1962), he comes back to it at the end of the 1960s and right at the beginning of the 1970s to give them, throughout the slow construction of his formulae of sexuation, its full logical extension to his provocative affirmation according to which '*il n'y a pas de rapport sexuel*': 'there is no sexual *rapport*'.[1]

A critical reading of these formulae requires an opening to the formal aspect of the difference between the sexes thanks to which, ever since the biblical disposition, the questions of the same and the difference relatively to man and woman are regulated. A brief glimpse of the quarrel about the universals in the Middle Ages allows it to be seen how, by wanting to describe the sexes in their difference, we remain caught up in the nets of an impossible coupling between a discreet conception where there are separated and form two essences and a conception in which we pass without a rupture from the one to the other and when there is never anything but something of the existence of the relative (these formal constraints remain active in Freud and Lacan). This is the object of the first chapter.

The approach of the Lacanian formulae also presupposed that one appreciates in their detail those of the tensions present in this teaching which led him to juggle with classical logic in order to subvert it with its ambition to universality. The invention, at the turn of the 1960s, of the object described as **o** and of its very curious quality of 'partial' object (in the sense that it would not maintain any '*rapport*' with any unity whatsoever) demanded that one should conceive of such a non-*rapport* and that one should venture towards the writing of a logical disequilibrium capable of taking in charge the shaky bipartition of the sexes. To do this, in his struggles with the all of the universal (and therefore of the concept), Lacan had to take this support on a use of the particular affirmative proposition that classical logic, hypnotised on this point by Aristotle, rejected into the margins of its treatises, and which corresponds to the ambiguity of most tongues with respect to the partitive 'some'. In general, the meaning of this term is restrictive: if the candidate has received 'some' votes, it is clear that he has not been elected, that he has not had all of them or even a simple majority. On the contrary, if, as a logician, I form the particular affirmative proposition 'some A are B', Aristotle pushes me to think that I am making there only a particular instantiation of the universal affirmative 'all A are B'. According to the implicit argument 'whoever can do the more can do the less', if all are so, some A are so also. It then follows, in accordance with the regulated ballet of propositions, that the affirmative and negative universals are contrary to one another.

By promoting the not-all, Lacan is making a play against Aristotle (and against Kant, at the same time), not by betting at the start on some property or other of feminine sexuality, but in making a choice of the restrictive particular, the one that means 'some, but not all'. In this case, by reason of the same formal constraints, the affirmative and negative particulars are equivalent (if some say yes, but not all, then it is also true that some others do not say yes). But it follows, preceding all, that since the universals ought to contradict their opposing particulars, and since the latter are equivalent, the universals are also. Here, common sense complains and prefers, like Aristotle, that they should be contrary and that the negative of the affirmative 'all say yes' should be 'all say no' and not 'there is not one that say does not yes' (we will see that in detail a little further, studying the different logical squares these universals belong to).

Lacan, for his part, holds very strongly, since his entry into the affair in 1962, that the negative universal should be understood in that way, as emptied of every element: this 'not one that . . .', he takes literally (with the help of Charles Sanders Peirce) in order to install there a nothing which he intends to be different to that of Freud or to that of Hegel, a nothing in agreement with the no being (*pas-d'être*) that he requires of his subject, represented by a signifier for another signifier. In all this, there is a coherence that the passage of the seminars hides and that must be reconstructed by setting aside sometimes the interpretation that Lacan himself proposes in order to give a quick meaning to his formulae. This is the object of the second chapter.

Because of having taken its support on an acceptance of the particular affirmative proposition which objects to the universal of the same quality, such an arrangement of the sexes, upsets the idea that one might have of a 'psychoanalytic' clinic. If one holds in effect that the affirmation of an existence goes against the concept under which it is put, we have to say good-bye to clinical vignettes and the other little accounts that the psychological world of today dotes on, where cases come in an exemplary way to be placed under the auspices of a theory more obsessed by its own transmission than by its uncertain and clashing relationship with practice. Contrary to appearances, these vignettes bear very little witness to the aforesaid practice in the measure that they pretend, above all, to illustrate a theoretical point of view that is judged to be too abstract. We then try to show in detail how this vignette style cheerfully shares in a relationship to the universality of the concept which transforms analytic knowledge into a psychology that is all the more unwelcome because it has far too much elbow room. Inversely, however conceptual it may be, the teaching of Lacan almost constantly fails to meet up with this naive functioning of universality in which the cases are only there to be put under concepts that unflinchingly await them. The universality of the concept – which there is no question of doing without – is regularly led by him to the point where it finds itself damaged, ruined even, not by accident but by the facts of language with which all thought including the most formal is exercised. The subject which is deduced from language and from its hold on a body in no way falls under the concept, not even that of subject. Here is something that escapes all psychopathologists, even indeed when they might think they are putting Lacanian concepts to work. That would be the object of the third chapter.

Finally, to show by a precise example how Lacan takes to task the concept and its object, I proposed to closely follow the affair, set up by him from one end to the other, of the unicity of the Borromean knot. Is there, yes or no, a single knot throughout the innumerable presentations that one can give of it? If yes, it will be possible, by means of some ad hoc definition, to have supported by this object well located in its positivity the sexual non-*rapport* which presents for its part the disadvantage of all negative appellations: one knows what it denies, but one does not know for all that what it is. And if not, if, in the end, there is not one such object, but several, with the impossibility of knowing which is the good one, we will have to abandon the support that *non-rapport* found in the knot, which Lacan recognises as true on 9 January 1979, at the quasi-end of his journey. This scholastic exercise deserved to be called a scolion.

Note

1 *Note from the author*: The expression is usually rendered into English as 'There is no sexual relationship'. Unfortunately, this is the source of a serious misunderstanding in the extent that Lacan never suggested that there is no sexual intercourse, of course. Using the ambiguity of the French word *rapport* he held, all along the last 10 years of his teaching, that from a Freudian point of view, 'man' and 'woman' must be conceived of as incommensurable the one to the other, without any possibility to establish a 'rapport' between them (mostly in the mathematical sense of the word). This is why, throughout this book, I discard the deceiving *relationship* in favour of the French *rapport* to slow the comprehension of the English reader on this tricky point.

1

THE LOGIC OF THE SEXUAL FAULT

That the sexes are two constitutes perhaps the most mysterious of certitudes, which divides in the most intimate way because it forces the path to a double regime of truth: yes, man and woman do indeed belong to the same species, the one called human (at the same time as they constitute, of course, the human genus [the French *genre* is translated as *genus* or *gender* in English]), but are they not so radically different from one another that one might believe that there exists between them a difference in the pure state, as decisive as irreducible? To the point that one takes up again the same word gender (*genre*) to differentiate, in the species, two classes of individuals, man/woman, whose union is crucial for the perpetuation . . . of the human genus! How can a genus be composed of a single species, which itself is divided into two genders? Homonomy! It will be said that the first *genre* does not have the same meaning as the second! And to be sure, it must indeed be so, but might there not be here an opportunity to envisage sexual difference in the logical and classificatory register in which it has been always expressed?

A metaphysical incest

God himself would seem to have made a mess of the affair, if one is to believe the short and enigmatic passage of Genesis I, 27, according to which '[s]o God created man in his image, in the image of God he created him; male and female he created him' and the much more complex operation that we can read just a little further on in Genesis II, 18–24:

18 Then the Lord God said, it is not good that the man should be alone; I will make him a helper as his partner.
19 So out of the ground the Lord God formed every animal of the field and every bird of the air and brought them to the man to see what he would call them: and whatever the man called every living creature that was its name.

20 The man gave names to all the cattle and to the birds of the air, and to every animal of the field: but for the man there was not found a helper as his partner.
21 So the Lord God caused a deep sleep to fall upon the man, and he slept; then he took one of his ribs and close up its place with flesh.
22 And the rib that the Lord God had taken from the man he made into a woman and brought her to the man.
23 Then the man said this at last is bone of my bones and flesh of my flesh; this one shall be called woman, for out of man this one was taken.
24 Therefore a man leaves his father and his mother and clings to his wife and they become one flesh.
25 And the man and his wife were both naked and were not ashamed.[1]

In Genesis I, 27 we witnessed a co-creation, man and woman emerging in parity, (almost) at the same time, without any logical advantage of the one over the other, scarcely a brief consecutiveness in the narrative; in Genesis II, 18–24, on the contrary, an order is put in place, which will serve throughout the millennia to justify the macho and religious patriarchies that we know.

If the woman is said here to proceed from the man, who was the first on the scene, it is, first of all, the guarantee the unicity of the genus. For in starting from the idea according to which every human individual comes from two parents, one is led to think of the origin of the species as a swarming.[2] Now, however little one might wish inversely to think of the origin as a principle, it is, on the contrary, imperative to pose a first term, as Aristotle himself invites us to (*Metaphysics a 1*) by affirming that for every genus, there exists an initial term, the principle of a series of elements that fall under the dominion of the genus.

The source alone – in this case, man – reduplicated in the woman fashioned by God gives a locus and a place for sexual difference and not, of course, the reverse; otherwise, it would have been necessary to make of this very difference the principle that would have held the entire genus under its dependency. Genesis II, 18–24, unfolds this progression from the one to the two then to the multiple, by affirming this time monogeneity, the engendering by a single one of his future partner and no longer a primordial couple (as in Genesis I, 27), which would have threatened the unicity of the genus and incurs a major risk: that man and woman might be conceived as two species within a same genus.

This would have been untenable since two species (save for the rarest of exceptions) cannot procreate, while man and woman are there biblically for that: to engender, to perpetuate the genus. It is necessary therefore for them to constitute only a single species, and hardly are they two, then they fold back into a single flesh, which is better understood if it is said in advance, as is the case of this very brief text, that the one is 'flesh of the flesh' of the other.

For copulation is not enough to organise such a logical and textual mystery: What is required so that the union of the principle (the man) and of what had then extracted from the principle (the woman) might produce something of the one? Nothing less than what Olivier Boulnois, in his article 'Un et un font un', names '*un inceste métaphysique: le principe doit s'unir à ce dont il est le principe pour se réunir en une seule unité*' (a metaphysical incest: the principle must unite itself with what he is the principle of in order to be reunited in a single unity).[3] To think through something so daring, the medieval theologians did not to be sure lack the means since the divine and the human, this irreducible duality, were found united in Christ, the one whose double nature in no way damages unity. But these same theologians, in order to sustain and, above all, to transmit conceptions so austere and rebellious to common sense, were obliged to support themselves more and more on authors – philosophers, logicians – which provided them with the tools for such an operation. This is where the story becomes complicated.

Nevertheless, it is worth the trouble to pause on the very long duration in the course of which there were forged the systems of thought which, still today, organise in an underhand way our reflections (and often our reflexes) on sex and gender. Thanks to the renewal of medieval studies, one can follow the business fairly closely, especially by finding support on the works of Alain de Libera[4] Inasmuch as he has been able to distinguish and to sort out the threads of a history that was too teleological, in too much of a hurry to find in the text what it already knew it was looking for.

The entry into the quarrel

Speaking about genus, species, difference, proper or accident, could not be done throughout the quasi-millennium that is gathered together under the name of the Middle Ages without referring oneself, in one way or another, to Porphyr's *Isagogue* since Boethius,[5] the teacher of the whole body of the learned for centuries, had begun with that: a commentary of this *Isagogue*, this text which served as an introduction to Aristotle before (and even after) the massive arrival of the latter via the Arab world. We find ourselves here immediately caught up in a curious enfilade: every medieval student began by plunging into the ready of the commentary that Boethius had done of Porphyr's *Isagogue*, a little text itself written around 270 CE by way of an introduction of Aristotle's text on the *Categories*. This, judged not without reason to be too difficult, in effect, called out for a commentary and, at the request of his friend Chrysaorios, Porphyr, who had studied at Athens and rejoined Plotinus in Rome (in 298 CE, after the death of the master, he published the *Enneades*), took on the task of editing some pages in which there would be presented the essentials of the Aristotelian text.

Let us forget for the moment Boethius and his own personal equation in order to better grasp the chasm between Aristotle and Porphyr in the measure that the famous quarrel about the Universals – about which I am here making the hypothesis that it continues to weigh heavily in the current debates about the sexes – came to birth there. Given the destiny of these few lines, we may as well read them attentively:

1 Since it is necessary, my dear Chrysaorios, for receiving the teaching relative to Aristotle's categories, to know what is (1) a genus, (2) a difference, (3) a species,

(4) a property, and (5) an accident, and since in order to give definitions for what concerns division as well as demonstration this study is useful, I will give you a short presentation on this subject, striving to go through, in brief, in the form of an introduction, what is found among the oldest authors, while all the time abstaining from entering into questions that are too profound, and only touching in a measured way on the easiest.

2 First of all, concerning the genus and the species, the question as to whether (1) they exist or indeed whether they only consist in pure concepts (2) or, supposing that they exist, whether they are bodies or incorporeal, and (3) in the last case, if they are separated or indeed if they exist in sensible things and in relationship with them – these are questions of which I will avoid speaking, because they represent a more profound research and because they call for another examination, that would be much longer.[6]

It is therefore by wanting to avoid 'questions that are too profound' that Porphry produces a sort of algorithm that is going to function as a formidable *topos*. Generations of teachers will transmit to generations of students this commonplace which draws all its power from the fact of being presented as a crossroads between Plato's realism and Aristotle's conceptualism. From the first point, if one chooses to consider that genera really exist,[7] the way is open to Platonic realism, according to which there exist before all separate forms in which singular individuals share; if one opts for a conception of the genus as a pure, conceptual entity which permits to gather by means of thought individuals that possess the same features, in order to constitute a class, then we find ourselves fully on the side of Aristotle.

But what divides also allows better than anything else to reunite, to articulate, to nuance, to intricate the systems of which each one presents advantages and not a few disadvantages. And this all the more that from the second point – whether if these genera really exist are they bodies or incorporeal? – here, in a single stroke, there is introduced the other great philosophical family, Stoicism, about which A. de Libera shows the degree to which it forms part of Porphyr's baggage, at several levels and in different ways.

The third of Porphyr's problems finally – if the genera are incorporeal, are they to be situated in sensible things or outside of them? – takes up again in a more subtle fashion the great Plato/Aristotle opposition on the question of formal ontology: Is the universal a separate form, or a form that is immanent in the sensible?

With this, this text functioned not alone as the required introduction to the *Categories* but as the minimal questionnaire starting from which there were deployed the systems (Platonism, Aristotelianism, Stoicism) that every teacher must learn, compare, and evaluate in order to be able to teach. This germinal aspect, drawn together in a simple form, was what gave its importance to this text of which Etienne Gilson asked himself already in 1942 'how could such an anodyne text have served as a starting point for such imposing metaphysical constructions which, from Boethius to the Renaissance, excited the most powerful minds'.[8]

Another point is here likely to attract our attention: nothing happened for five centuries. It is only at the turning point of the 11th and the 12th centuries that there explodes the quarrel of the universals, in other words – a remarkable thing – well before the arrival of the Aristotelian and Platonic corpus, at a time when the erudite have still nothing to get their teeth into than fragments of Greek texts: a fragment of the Timaeus for Plato, and the two first treatises of the *Organon* for Aristotle (the *Categories* and *De interpretatione*). It is therefore not confronted with the complexity, the riches, and the ambiguity of the Greek texts soon transmitted along the Arab route that the translation of Porphyr's *Isagogue* by Boethius had taken on a sudden relief. The historians of philosophy lose themselves here in conjectures about the veritable cause of the debate, already fully attested by Abelard (1079–1142), hence the problem: To what should we attribute such a time of incubation? What happened for Porphyr's lines translated by Boethius inflamed and opposed minds when, for such a long time, no one saw any malice in it? I am happy to hold with the hypothesis of Alain de Libera, even if the way it begins is very prudent:

> It is probably, that here as elsewhere, trinitarian theology played a determining role. It is the mystery of the Greek definition of three persons as '*tres usie, id est tres substantie*' which, together with the question of whether the three Persons were 'only one thing (*una tantaum res*) or three distinct things (*tres res per se*)', gave rise to the response of Roscelin de Compiegne, denounced by Anselm, according to which, it was really necessary that the Father, the Son and the Spirit were three distinct things if one wanted to avoid the theologically dangerous conclusion, that 'the Father was incarnated at the same time as the Son'. By this, the fragments of Aristotelian ontology and semantics which the higher Middle Age had as its disposition were mobilised, and by unexpected paths the question 'what is substance?' about which Aristotle had made, in his *Metaphysics*, the question eternally pursued, had effectively rediscovered a second youth. . . . The reading of the *Isagogue* then changed its status. From a simple index of definitions, Porphyr's manual became an index of questions.[9]

The mystery of the union in the difference, of the unity of a plurality, of the belonging of an individual to his genus, would then, first of all, have been divine in the measure that, in these regions and according to the options that one took up, one went very quickly from the pulpit to the stake. Here there was an urgency in settling what the majority of current affairs willingly left in the shadows. And therefore, even before the mass of Aristotelian and Platonic texts unfurled, Roscelin de Compiegne[10] had, in a way, opened the quarrel by supporting extreme options.

The first steps

He claims in effect that universal terms (like *man*) are only *flatus vocis*, or again vocalisations, words which do not call for or designate any existent reality, which leads him in accordance with proper logic to maintain that no thing is made up of parts, in the sense that there does not exist any thing which collects together other things. For us, post-Bourbakiens who have swallowed whole the intangible truth according to which a set is more than the sum of its parts – therefore exists apart from them – takes our breath away a little. The apparent absurdity of the thesis only makes it more attractive: no all exists because it would be necessary to think of it as outside the sum of its parts and thus to tip over into the opinion that there exists substantially things that go beyond the collections of objects of which they are constituted and therefore are not any object. In this way, Roscelin responds to Pierre Abelard, who criticises him on this point, that 'once the part that makes the man has been taken away, he should be called not Peter, but Peter incomplete'; otherwise, it would be necessary to believe in the existence of a thing which would remain the same in the case of the removal of one of its parts.[11] What leads Roscelin to enunciate his second thesis, according to which only *voces*, names or vocal sounds, exist, and the singular things referred to by these names, insofar as they possess qualities that do not separate them, that they are 'alls whose parts remain solidary', in short, that they are all like pebbles, each of which would bear the same name.

For Abelard, on the contrary, names are attributed to things indirectly, in function of their signification, in other words, in function of the essence of the thing, which persists whether the parts are all present or not. This essence is not necessarily an independent thing to which the name would univocally refer (in this, he follows his master against the future realists who hold mordicus in the effective real existence of Platonic ideas, of separated form), but it allows us to think, between the object as all and the name, of a third articulation situated at the level of a signification, which is not confused either with the *flatus vocis* of the name or with the object which serves as reference.

These are, from the first steps of the quarrel, two semantics which are confronted: the one of *signification*, with Abelard and his concern to maintain separated the question of the essence and that of the all, and the other of *reference* with Roscelin, who, for his part, only understands a direct link between the sound of a word and its reference.[12]

Without even going any further, it becomes possible to distinguish between two alls, which allows the arguments like those of Roscelin to be settled from the 13th century on but which also prove that one cannot work in this type of problem without possessing at least two notions of all-compassing unity. Already at the time of Roscelin, a certain Garland-the-counter made a difference between the 'universal all' and the 'integral all'. The first, defined as superior and substantial, presented itself as a unity composed of parts described as subjective, themselves thought of as what is inferior to the universal; the universal all corresponded therefore to the present-day conception of class which subsumes, comprehends, includes a number x of elements that one will describe to go quickly as detachable. The integral whole, for its part, is the singular thing, the subject part of the universal all, composed of real parts that cannot be detached from their all without adulterating it (while removing an element of the class does not threaten it as a class). We see that Roscelin error consisted in wanting to confuse these two alls (these two ones) and that Abelard was able to criticise and rectify his master on the basis of their distinction.

The Abelardian critique was also brought to bear against his other master, Guillaume de Champeaux, who supported the existence 'in the things that differ among themselves, of a substance essentially the same, the material essence of singular beings in which it is: one in itself and diverse only by the forms of beings put under it'.[13] In this optic, not only does the foundational substance of the genus really exist, but it also is present in each one of the elements that it collects in this way. Each man is therefore clearly singular, but these singular men, distinct in themselves, 'are a same being in man (*in homine*), namely that they do not differ in the nature of humanity'. They are therefore 'singular by reason of their distinction' but are 'said to be universals by reason of the non-difference *and* of their conjunction in a same resemblance'. The quarrel of universals takes off from this final *and*, which, in its way, goes back to Socrates theses in the *Menon* (which Guillaume had in no way at his disposal).

Is everything that is not different for all that alike? Socrates's proof is brought to bear for its part on bees: since nothing distinguishes one bee *qua* bee from another bee *qua* bee, it is, first of all, on the perception of the non-difference between individuals that one will conclude to their belonging to the same species, and not by a first recognition, in each individual, of a something identical. Specific identity, in the empirical and epistemological perspective of Socrates, comes from the absence of difference, but this non-difference is not, in itself, any being apart, does not enjoy therefore any ontological weight inversely to the other option which would make exist first of all an identical part in each one, thus reducing specific identity to being nothing more than a necessary consequence of the effective presence in each individual of a minimum common to all, in which from then on the notion of species and of genus take refuge.

This algorithm traversed the centuries and divided minds. Because he did not have to choose in this way between an extreme Platonic realism and the absurdities of his master Roscelin, Abelard had to support this *semantic of signification* thanks to his invention of the *status*. This term is his alone. Only an untimely anachronism would make of it our post Saussurian 'signified'. Abelard's approach here is more disturbing but by that very fact is richer: since everything is singular, it is itself and cannot be anything else. *Exit* the idea, fundamental for the realists, that a thing could be predicated of another thing, that a specific identity could reside as such in the singular identity of an individual (and that therefore resemblance would take precedence over non-difference, since it would come from the effective presence of the same presence among individuals that otherwise are different). Only a noun, according to Abelard, 'can serve as a predicate for several subjects taken one by one'. Only a universal word, and not a thing, can fulfil this function. We are, alas, so quickly persuaded that we no longer take the measure of Abelard's audacity in inserting in this way, between singular things and the pure *flatus vocis* of the name, this *status*, this state which flirts with the Platonic idea (and allows it to be thought that God possesses the status of every thing even before it exists – creation is saved) without conferring on it the slightest real existence. But this invention also sets aside the concept because it is a matter less of what will be thought than of what is said by the universal words *man*, *animal*, and so on. When, in Genesis II, 18–20, Adam pronounces the names of the species which process before him, it is not under the name of founding its concept but of producing its Abelardian *status*, in other words, to make each species subsist in the tongue and not in thought.

The name of 'woman': where to place the difference?

How then comprehend, along this vein, verse 23? This time again, Adam pursues his work as a giver of names when, waking up from the torpor that God had made fall on him in order to operate this costal subtraction, he says: 'She will be called woman for it is from a man that she has been taken'. Here is a new animal that has been presented to him and now that he's got going he names the one with whom from the following verse on he would no longer be but 'one flesh'. What is here his linguistic operation? Origen, in his commentary on the Gospel of Matthew (14, 16–17), recalls the Hebrew text the better to articulate the terminological differences from Genesis I, 27:

> 'Man' is here designated by the word is, and 'male' by the word Zachar; and again woman by the word ISSA, and the female by the word Ankeba.[14]

Zachar and *Ankeba*, 'male' and 'female', are words which are opposed without having very much in common, as in their extemporaneous apparition in Genesis I, 27; inversely, in Genesis II, 23, ISSA is presented as a direct derivation of IS, which is why Latin in this place uses the word *virago* to maintain the obvious community of linguistic root between IS and ISSA. These considerations form part of the patrimony of commentators of every epoch, as is testified by these lines of Dominique Grima,[15] who, in the first half of the 14th century, glossed Genesis II, 23 by taking right away Adam's voice:

> *And this woman*, formed from me, will be called, by her proper name which I impose on her, mannesse (*hommesse*) and this appropriately since she has been taken from man. Manesse [virago] is in effect a name drawn from the name man as a material taken from a material. This denomination figures in the Hebrew text: in effect, man is called ish in Hebrew, woman isha (the same relationship between manesse and man). This name was the proper name of the first woman. Now one calls manesse any woman who acts like a man. The syncopated form of virago is virgo [virgin], as Pierre le Mangeur says. That is why, as long as they preserve the integrity of their birth, women are called virgins; subsequently, once they are fractured they are called mulieres [women], for as it were 'softening the hero', namely men. In the same manner, Adam was the name of the first man, as le Mangeur says, but now it is a common name.[16]

This passage, from the proper to the common, leads back to the Porphyrien *Categories* (genus, species, difference, property, accident) with which the higher Middle Age tried to resolve these problems and allows us now to advance into some of the arcana of the quarrel fortified by this sexual difference as a viaticum as it were. It is here also that we rediscover the personal equation of Boethius.

Like every translator, he cannot avoid taking sides, however transparent he may want to be in his task. In this way, at the first difficulty, he leans openly, even though silently, to Aristotle's side in order to support the idea that genera and species cannot be substances using a reasoning present in *Metaphysics Z* according to which, since genera and species are simultaneously common to a plurality of individual things, they themselves do not possess any numerical unity that is valid for every singular being. Not being singular in this sense, they cannot have the degree of existence of a substance.

But at the same time – and this without the help of Aristotle or Plato – they cannot be either be situated only in the intellect (which we for our part imagine too easily), because 'every active intellect is made starting from something which is its subject'. No one can have in his mind something that he has not, first of all, had in his senses and conceptualising something which is supposed to be nowhere is ruled out. From that comes a double and untenable requirement: it must be affirmed that genera and species are indeed something in reality (*in rerum veritate*) without being for all that substances and that moreover they are indeed in the intellect but not as empty concepts that would refer to nothing in reality.

Boethius succeeds in doing so by finding support on the mechanism of perception as it was conceived by Alexander of Aphrodise: according to the latter, sensations present to the soul in an incorporeal form are things which in themselves are corporeal. If therefore the spirit, pursues Boethius, 'can distinguish what the senses transmit to it as mixed up (*confuse*) and attached (*conjuncta*) to bodies, and in this way to contemplate (*speculari*) and see the incorporeal nature by itself, without the bodies in which it is mixed up (*concreta*)', then the same spirit has the power to consider and contemplate genera and species 'by separating the incorporeals that it receives combined (*permixta*) to bodies'.[17]

This crucial operation is called *abstraction*, a noun that of itself is too polysemic for us to be satisfied with it. The Middle Ages distinguished, in effect, *mathematical abstraction* (which aims at the production of abstract beings, forms grasped by mathematical activity); *mystical abstraction* which, according to the Pseudo-Dionysus the Aeropagite, allows the Christian to raise himself up by thought from the world of beings to the superessential (on the model of the sculptor who brings out from the block of marble the statue that was latent in it); and, finally, the abstraction that will be called *epistemological*, the only one that interests us here.

By *abstractive induction* is understood going from elements held to be similar to their gathering together under a same notion (therefore under the same name), but in what way? We will not be too surprised to rediscover here two families of thinkers as close as they are opposed on this sore point of the quarrel. One side are partisans of the fact that a name permits resemblances to be grasped, to regroup under the same *flatus vocis* and a same *status* numerical singular beings. As A. de Libera points out in the article 'Abstraction' of the *Dictionnaire du Moyen Âge*,[18] this conception extends as far as Locke who, in his *Essay on Human Understanding*, still wrote: 'The grouping of things under names is the work of understanding, which takes the occurrence of the similitude that it observes among them to forge general abstract ideas'. But others privilege a different path: to neutralise these singular features in a numerically singular individual, in order to produce the abstract type which will no longer present anything other than the common features likely to gather together the plurality of singular individuals liable for an identical operation of abstraction. The first based themselves on the existence of an already-present resemblance which it is only a matter of picking out of the intellect (our modern notion of class); the others produce non-difference by setting aside all the features that founded the difference divisible between the singular individuals (by producing the type from which the genus flowed, as in the case of Adam). The first perceive directly the resemblance between the individuals; for the second, this resemblance is not a sensible given but a construction *per via di levare*, as one goes from a triangle traced out in the sand to the abstract idea of triangle by removing its particularities to get to its 'type'.

On property and difference

These subtleties will appear to belong to a different age if one loses sight of the current debate on sexual difference, but the feminist wave and the conception become banal today of the equality of the sexes have not freed us as much as we might believe from the infernal question of difference in the common belonging to the human race. Quite the contrary: if one does not approach in however little a way to these medieval exercises in disputation, one strongly risks being precipitated towards a conception of sexual difference which misses out on the logical problem on which it reposes.

The latter, in effect, puts to work so directly the most basic elements of our understanding that we must lose hope of possessing by ourselves the conceptual tools which would allow us to describe it correctly. Psychoanalysis does not offer at this point any privileged point of view, however detailed may be the theoretical and clinical knowledge that it offers us on this chapter. One of the rare possibilities available returns therefore to make vacillate our most natural conceptions (those that we have learned in primary school) by confronting them with others.

If one enunciates the problem in an apparently minimal form, one comes up against an irreducible duality: on the one side, the man/woman opposition is perfectly discrete, every subject is either one or the other and only falls under one category and it alone;[19] on the other side, they are two qualities that ceaselessly interpenetrate according to a gradient which leads from the most manly man to the most womanly woman while passing through all the intermediary combinations. Therefore, sexual difference shamelessly mixes two qualities that understanding holds to be heterogeneous: the discreet and the continuous.

These data have become easier to enunciate since the work of Thomas Laqueur *La Fabrique du sexe*,[20] which establishes with all historical clarity this duplicity (more than duality), inherent to the sexes. That our unshakeable conviction, according to which there exist two sexes morphologically, histologically, genetically differentiateable, had been preceded by a very long period where there only existed, for each and every one, one sex unequally shared by each gender, here is something that even today creates the effect of a scoop. Naturally, when one approaches it, this so-called historical succession contains a whole complex overlapping: the theory of the two sexes has always been there, more or less, and the thought of a single sex, however damaged it has been by science, continues to irrigate many discourses. There remains, however, the idea of the same mental obstruction, in styles of thought (*episteme*) almost impervious with respect to one another, with regard to this duality that people try in vain to support, sometimes on a 'proper' (what is man is in no way woman and vice versa), sometimes on an 'accident' coming to alter in different ways subjects identical apart from that.

Freud

The Freudian discovery is inscribed in this long history, especially with the texts of 1923 that establish the very subtle business of the phallic phase. Freud puts in place there a kind of trunk that is common to the boy and to the girl, already present in the *Three Essays on Theory of Sexuality* of 1905, that rests in fact on the conception of one libido referring only to one sex (the masculine):

> Indeed, if we were able to give a more definite connotation to the concepts of masculine and feminine, it would even be possible to maintain that libido is invariably and necessarily of a masculine nature, whether it occurs in men or in women and irrespectively of whether its object is a man or a woman.[21]

Like the little boy, the little girl discovers masturbatory pleasure, the one playing with her clitoris and the other with his penis. So far, it's a draw. A first difference is discovered starting from the reciprocal site that each obtains of the genitals of the other: the little boy pretends (*dixit* Freud) to have seen nothing: 'He begins by showing irresolution and lack of interest', because what he sees would run the strong risk of giving weight to the threat of castration that he has received, perceived, but that up to now he had not taken seriously. For the little girl, it is quite the contrary: 'She makes her judgment and her decision in a flash. She has seen it and knows that she is without it and wants to have it'.[22]

She is therefore going to enter into the Oedipus complex by the castration complex and begins to want a child from the father as a substitute for this absent penis, while the little boy, if all goes well from a Freudian point of view, will emerge for his part from his Oedipus complex by this same castration complex which, by incarnating the narcissistic threat to this part of his own body, will manage to make his incestuous libidinal cathexes fall back. To save his precious penis, he will let go of his mother (unless by simply repressing all of that, which opens wide for him the door to neurosis).

Such at least is the story that Freud launches from 1903 and re-orchestrates in 1923. The success of this conception, like the violence of the attacks of which it has been, of which it is still, the object bears witness to its insertion into a multi-secular problematic. The libido theory, however novel it was in many aspects, moulded itself also onto complete antiquities and in all of that deserves our attention. From the chapter on the differentiation between men and women in his *Three Essays*, Freud notes three distinct senses of the opposition of the concepts of masculine and feminine:

> It is essential to understand clearly that the concepts of masculine and feminine, whose meaning seems so ambiguous to ordinary people are among the most confused that occur in science. It is possible to distinguish at least three uses. Masculine and feminine are used sometimes in the sense of activity and passivity, sometimes in a biological and sometimes again in a sociological sense. The first of these three meanings is the essential one and the most serviceable in psychoanalysis. When for instance libido was described in the text above as being masculine, the word is being used in this sense, for an instinct is always active even when it has a passive aim in view. The second, or biological meaning of masculine and feminine is the one whose applicability can be determined most easily. Here masculine and feminine are characterized by the presence of spermatozoa or ova respectively and by the functions proceeding from them . . . the third or sociological meaning receives its connotation from the observation of actually existing masculine and feminine individuals such observation shows that in human beings pure masculinity or femininity is not to be found either in a psychological or a biological sense.[23]

Twenty-two years later, the same words return when he writes to conclude his article on 'Some Psychical Consequences of the Anatomical Distinction between the Sexes':

> [A]ll human individuals as a result of the bi-sexual disposition and of cross-inheritance, combine in themselves both masculine and feminine characteristics, so that pure masculinity and femininity remain theoretical constructions of uncertain content.[24]

The formal configuration of the entities manipulated here to the point of having the merit, not of clarity, at least of duration. In this way, Freud is confronted with the duplicity evoked earlier: on the one side, with the biological *Bedeutung*, he looks for an instant as if he is holding with the male/female a couple in opposition which would present the high point of functional differentiation (ovum/spermatozoa); on the two other sides, psychological or sociological, all the mixed forms are conceivable.

A lesson: the sexes are only easily differentiable in the heart of the germinal cells, when meiosis has made them pass to the diploid stage (23 pairs of chromosomes) to the haploid stage (23 chromosomes) and that the all *x* ova henceforth offer themselves to an encounter with the spermatozoa that are sometimes all *x* sometimes all *y*. There perhaps one could speak, with precaution, of pure masculinity and of pure femininity. Afterwards . . . even if the chromosomic lottery is inevitably going to make foetal evolution tend towards the production of male XY or female XX cells, the somatic organisation, for its part, will no longer give up on an irreducible ambiguity. The biological rock of the 23rd chromosome will then come to support the imaginary of a difference that is completely potential, with its TDF gene carried by the little Y chromosome and held to be responsible for the masculine phenotype, while the female XX will henceforth give the appearance of being the strong sex, because of its homogeneity.

Freud did not know all this – even though one can think that he would have liked the double helix. But we must agree that this knowledge about the genetic forge of the human reinforces the common opinion on the idea of an irreducible difference, since we know it is inscribed in the microscopical innermost parts of each of ourselves. If, according to Freud's word echoing that of Napoleon, anatomy is destiny, what can we say then about genetics? Transvestites and transsexuals may push as far as they can the corporeal transformations that they want, but it is hard to see them entirely changing themselves, unless by falling once more into the problem of Theseus's boat, in which one comes to change the totality of the elements that compose it and as regards which one can ask if it is indeed still 'Theseus's boat'.[25] It is therefore necessary, not alone in practice but also in thought, to support the existence of separate male/female entities, even if only in the short time of the mitotic pre-encounter.

Thus, the content of the theoretical construction of pure masculinity and pure femininity is no longer as uncertain as in Freud's time – and nevertheless, I maintain that the setting has not fundamentally changed because of this, by reason of the permanence of logical and mental constraints. This blueprint according to which we isolate two entities that one would like to believe independent because science was able to locate them to name them, to separate them only stretches the two extremities between which there slides more than ever the ferret of sexual determination. We learn with surprise and amusement that one of the star dancers of the Beijing Opera was a former colonel in the Red Army and that, for more than a millennium, people were afraid of the usurpation of a Pope Joan:[26] all this goes to show that, in certitude, if it does not reign, at least it is always able to show the tip of its nose, since positions so marked sexually do not offer any trustworthy guarantee.

Therefore, Freud does not free himself from a figure of thought in which each and every one finds themselves engaged when it is a matter of going from the difference of the sexes to the existence of two sexes each well individuated. So the problem is henceforth established fairly clearly on the formal plane: Do the sexes exist only relative to one another; in the end, is sexual difference anything other than what Aristotle named a relative? Or, indeed, does each one of these sexes depend on a singular substance so that sexual difference would only be the consequence of this duality of substances? To delve more deeply into this formal aspect of the question it would be as well to turn towards a less charged relative than that of sexual difference: What is heat, and what is cold?

Absolute versus relative

Right away, one is tempted to respond that, as for light and shade or big and small, cold and heat are exclusive relative values, which are only defined in relationship to one another. Having conventionally posed what it is agreed to hold as hot, I will hold to be cold, in other words as less hot, everything that presents a lesser thermal agitation, and reciprocally. The more and the less, emblems of all the relatives, seem to reign as masters over cold and heat. But such is not the case always and everywhere.

Scarcely has one learned that heat is only a certain degree of agitation of matter than the omnipresence of the relative comes up against, in thermal matters, a ground value: the zero quite rightly called absolute, at –273.16 °C (or 0 °K). Since temperature measures the degree of movement of molecules vis a vis one another (in gasses and liquids, to be sure, but also in solids), the degree 0 corresponds to the state of absolute rest in which, not alone do the molecules no longer move but at which also the electrons would stop turning their kernel and around themselves (spin). Even though at the present time the record has been pushed to 10^{-10} °K, it is clear that there is no question of going beyond this limit: How go any further in rest when nothing is moving any longer?

Inversely, temperature knows no upper limit: if the agitation becomes too intense, the molecules break up, the atoms themselves are shattered into states described as plasmatic. If the energy is lacking to create states of matter that are still more intense in which the most elementary particles would lose their consistency, nothing prevents us from thinking about such a situation. Imagination, which encountered with rest a veritable wall in the progression towards a more cold, comes up against nothing of the sort on the side of the universal furnace (unless by thinking of infinite energies at the 0 time of the Big Bang. A difficult exercise).

At the same time, on the side of speed, general relativity has come, for its part also, to upset imagination and its natural taste for relatives, for the more or the less as far as you can see, by positioning an absolute upper limit: nothing can go faster than light. This new datum might appear just as mysterious as the absolute 0 in temperature, if reasoning did not come in the same way to support imagination in this maze: since what puts a break on movement is inertia, in other words, the mass of what is moving, nothing can go faster than what possesses a null mass. Now this is the case of the photon. Therefore, nothing can go faster than a photon. Certain relatives can tolerate therefore coming up against limiting values, sorts of asymptotes unreachable by definition and in that ready to incarnate stable points, foreign to variation, which in a continuous or discreet fashion, work on the relatives, in short ideal candidates to reaffirm the idea of substance: something that does not move and remains identical to itself, independently of the qualities that affect it and of the relations that it justifies.

But where is the hen; where is the egg? Must we think that there are, first of all, separate substances and that the relative only arrange a progressive distancing from this fixed given or that, inversely, there is only the relative more and less that provide us with our daily experience and that with that we construct (helped much more by reasoning than by intuition) entities that set bounds to these relatives?

Is there in this way, an equal ontological dignity, Man and Woman[27] *qua* separated entities, real posts between which each human being would slide as it were along a clothes line in order, finally, to be caught, at the whim of a capricious bisexuality? Or indeed are there only relatives, sexual difference as far as one can see, without ever managing to be hypostasised in these opposing blocks to which imagination alone exercises its wits, for its part, in practising an induction (doubtful in its principle) according to which the local truth (the sexual difference) is only the instantiation of a global truth (of an irreducible substantial duality)?

Lacan and inaccessibility

The incubation time of this question in Lacan's teaching is remarkable. For almost 15 years, even though going through the most diverse themes, we see him scarcely retouching the Freudian arrangement in the matter even while he redefines and subverts it in many of its points. The categories of man and woman just as indispensable in clinical descriptions as in the course of theoretical elaborations, scarcely calls for a direct questioning. We have to wait for the little text 'Directive Remarks for a Congress on Feminine Sexuality'[28] to appreciate his first cut at the question. It is outstandingly relative, in the sense that no nature come to define each of the sexual partners. The dominance of symbolic determinations requires that each one only finds its status in function of the other, indeed of the Other, which one single quotation will be enough to give a sense of:

> [C]astration cannot be deduced from development alone, since it presupposes the subjectivity of the Other *as the* locus of its law. *The otherness of sex is misrepresented by this alienation.* A man serves here as a relay in order that a woman should become this Other to herself, as she is to him.[29]

No question therefore of looking for some nature of each sex. The differences of functioning that are described – for example 'an enjoyment enveloped in its own contiguity' on the side of the woman and 'a desire that castration liberates in the male by giving him his signifier in the phallus'[30] on the side of man do not allow separate entities to be constructed; each one is so much made to respond to the other as least as much as to put into operation some specificity or other.

On the other hand, there is outlined a putting into relation of each speaking being with sexual enjoyment, without the latter undergoing the habitual bipartition which would have it that each sex has its own. Linked as it is to the phallus, when, with the appearance of the **o**-object, the latter progressively sees its quality of substantive vanishing in favour of its adjectival value, it ends up by being called 'phallic enjoyment'. There is here a direct echo of the Freudian assertion already encountered according to which there is only one type of libido, the male type, but this exclusivity was attached in Vienna to the idea of the libido as pure activity – the sign of a fatal confusion between the discrete definition of sex (Man/Woman) and its continuous definition (more or less active/more or less passive).

By not using this recourse to more and less which could not but mix up, in his eyes, the symbolic dimension and the imaginary dimension, Lacan found himself uneasy in supporting such a unicity of libido, while he ruled out the hypothesis (that he denounced in Jones) of 'to each sex its own enjoyment'. But how get out of such a tight corner? It is enough to pose such a question in order to see him, after an interval of some months, engaging himself in a curious maze on what one could call, enforcing a bit the feature, the number of enjoyments.

The first step does not have the merit of clarity. It takes place towards the end of one of the last sessions of the seminar . . . *Ou pire*, 10 May 1972, at the moment when Lacan finds himself led, for reasons that one does not right away perceive, to comment that the actual infinite, $\aleph_0$ is an 'inaccessible' in the sense that no summation or exponentiation of its subparts reaches it. And in this sense, it will be revelatory of the additional one (*un-en-plus*) that Lacan tracks as being what is realised in every operation of counting. He must feel that he is himself engaged in an awkward French oratorical situation, since he adds: 'To end I am going to make you sense in a quite simple form which is the following . . .'.

And to explain a property described as accessibility according to which a whole number would be called accessible if it could be constructed, either as the sum or as the exponentiation of (whole) numbers smaller than it. The 1, says Lacan, 'I sufficiently underlined that it is engendered from the fact that the 0 marks from lack', and in any case, having only a single antecedent, the rule of accessibility is not applied to it. It is only really posed with the 2. Now, with the 0 and the 1, however one combines them, one does not reach 2, while starting from 2, it is obvious that every number becomes accessible as the sum or the exponentiation any two of its predecessors. Here then the number 2 is proclaimed inaccessible. The reader of these lines may indeed be just as questioning as the listener of that time: Where then is Lacan trying to get to with these *ad hoc* properties? To be sure, he wants there to be understood the fact that the consideration of the real straight line [0, 1] hollows out between each whole number a numerical space where there is situated nothing less than the actual infinity and that therefore every whole number is like a $\aleph$ for its predecessor. But how does this consideration which looks so Bourbakienne touch him? Only the final lines of this session allow it to be understood:

> [W]hat is involved, and what I started from, is what is designed to suggest to you the utility of the fact that there is something of the 1, (in order) that you should be able to understand what is involved in this bipartition at every fleeting instant, this bipartition of the man and the woman: that every that

> is not man is woman one would tend to admit. But since the woman is not notall, why would everything that is not woman be man? This bipartition, this impossibility of applying, in this business of gender, something which is the principle of contradiction . . . , is what I am indicating to you as being what ought to allow the analyst to understand a little bit more.[31]

Only a work of approximation, to be read in the course of the following chapter, will allow us to read this strange not-all that collides with the woman. But what explodes already, at the level of the counting of the habitual couple Man/Woman, is a disequilibrium, which Lacan refers back to a stumbling of the principle of contradiction, which moreover trenches on the principle of the excluded third. In a first phase, he, in effect, makes not-man equivalent to woman, but denying woman (therefore, not [not man]), he does not come back to man. The reason why he sometimes invokes intuitionist logic since the latter, excluding the principle of the excluded third, does not hold as equivalent a term and the negation of its negation. But I doubt that it would be all that very useful to get any more involved in the functioning of intuitionist logic to read the formulae of sexuation, not before at least having gone through the classical aspects under which they are presented. The two sexes in his eyes do not share gender in such a way that, on the plane of extension, everything that is not to be put on one side is to be put on the other or vice versa: *exit* the Yin and the Yang and all the couples in opposition that claim in different cultures to rule by one and the same gesture the number of sexes and the logical meaning of contradiction of meaning.

In wanting to settle the question on the plane that he had brought out as symbolic, and in refusing the Freudian recourse to the imaginary of the active/passive tension, Lacan comes on the problem of the numeration of sexes: more than 1 but not 2. No means of acceding to the two, the second does not manage to close (*boucler*) its unity like the first, and therefore the count irresistibly stumbles. A year later, this formal problem re-emerges at the level of the counting of enjoyments.

Neither 1 nor 2

If Lacan was able, in effect, to use the term and the concept 'phallus' in a very accentuated way, the different writings that he produces for it in the course of the seminars suffice to guarantee its polyphony: *grand phi*, Φ, for the phallus described as symbolic and *little phi*, φ, for the imaginary phallus (sometimes put into a negative form as *minus phi*: $-\varphi$). It is, of course, a signifier but a signifier at the limit since it would be the only one to be able to signify itself; it is also sometimes an object; it also very special when it is described as 'metonymic'; in other words, it is the catastrophic point of the system so dear to structuralism, the chiasm that inverts all values. Now at the moment when Lacan sets out – very late – to pronounce on the duality Man/Woman, the substantive phallus tends to be effaced, becomes much less conceptually charged and becomes an adjective to qualify, sometimes a function (that we will study later), sometimes an enjoyment, THE enjoyment it must almost be said, about it, there is no room to doubt it. It is, in Lacan's eyes, that which, in the structure of the subject, is imposed because of language and determines that the human being cannot advance towards his satisfactions except by emerging himself in language. The human being, this *neotene*, this being so incomplete at his birth, post-partum, makes of language one of his principle organs and this organ enjoys. On this there is no hesitation: there is something that is called phallic jouissance. It strikes each and every one in that no one is a subject if he does not manage to produce himself as such in and by language, by participating in this enjoyment that articulates body and speech and definitively links sexual pleasure to the interplay of signifiers, of phonation and audition. The unicity proclaimed about the Freudian libido finds here in Lacan its direct echo, in this universality of phallic enjoyment. But as is often the case with him, taking it up again is followed by a subversion. Might it be, he asks himself on 13 February 1973, that there had been another enjoyment? The question is by no means innocent since, even on the side of the Freudian analysts of the time, there are quite a few who think quite openly that it is so, Jones at their head (others more discreetly).

The merit of the expression 'phallic enjoyment' is that it does not bring about by itself any division. It is valid, one can begin to say it in this way, for every speaking being, without, first of all, asking either its sex or its gender. Such a universality poses of itself the question of its pertinence, of the breadth of its extension: Is it really the only one to reign over this domain called by Lacan enjoyment, a direct equivalent for which one might search almost in vain in Freud? In the Freudian corpus, in effect, *Lust* is only pleasure, which obeys its principle. The German word *Genus*, which might be translated as 'enjoyment', is very rare and has no conceptual value. There remains the beyond of the pleasure principle, which Lacan translates for his part by 'enjoyment', hence the strangeness of the question that he poses on 13 February 1973: Might it be that there are two 'beyond'?

The response that he gives plays, first of all, on the ambiguities of the French tongue and grammar, which offer him the shelter of the protasis and the apodosis (he himself employs these terms during his seminar). The protasis is a conditional subordinate placed at the head of the sentence, necessarily followed by its apodosis, which is nothing other than the principle proposition: *s'il l'exige, je partirai*; *si vous n'arrivez pas à l'heure, je ne vous attendrai pas.*[32] In function of an imperious concordance of tenses in this respect, the presence of the protasis calls on the future of the apodosis, and the imperfect, the conditional. Now the imperfect can have just by itself a very hypothetical value, already underlined by Lacan for different ends: *un instant plus tard, et la bombe éclatait*, a sentence which does not say by itself whether the bomb has exploded or if it has simply almost done so but that nothing of the kind happened.

'*S'il y en avait une autre, il le faudrait pas que ce soit celle-là*'. Here we have enunciated the regime of the existence of an enjoyment which would be other than phallic. Lacan hastens to point out the equivocation of the final *celle-là*: Which one? The other whose existence the protasis presupposes or 'the one from which we started to designate this other as other',[33] therefore the phallic? This stealthy vacillation between the deictic value, which refers back to the situation of the enunciating, and the anaphoric value, which refers back to the antecedents in the enunciation itself, is quickly settled in favour of the latter: Supposing that there had been one other than phallic, then it would not be appropriate,[34] but to whom and to what? To the act of saying, 'The aforesaid enjoyment is repressed because it is not appropriate that it should be said, and this precisely for the reason that the act of saying can be nothing other than the following – as enjoyment, it is not suitable'.[35]

This non-appropriateness is nevertheless far from being sufficient for Lacan, who is seeking here to tickle something much more subtle than the representation incompatible with the ego, on which Freud had based the concept of secondary repression. This enjoyment, in effect, is nothing that exists and which would be such that it should be repressed; the business must be pushed to the point where its non-existence is sustained. Taking support from the logical operator of implication, present in the protasis/apodosis couple, Lacan argues from the fact that a false antecedent can very well lead to a true consequent, and that in this case the implication remains valid, and therefore: 'It is false that there is an other, which does not prevent what follows being true, namely that it would not be necessary that it should be this one'.[36]

One could scarcely refine any more the degree of supposition. This indirectly evokes the Descartes of the *Principes de la philosophie*[37] but comes back above all to affirm an inexistence, a movement of enunciation of which Lacan knows for a fact the degree of paradox that it involves since the simple fact of affirming gives to the object of affirmation this minimum of existence that language confers on everything that it brings to the act of saying. That the reference may be empty, as in the case of squared circles, does not for all that make them purely and simply inexist, in the measure that the signification allows there to be welcomed beings as well as non-beings, it is, in any case, the reason for which one sees Lacan swerve rapidly, in the same page 56 of *Encore*, on being and non-being: 'Well then, that non being should not be, it must not be forgotten that it is added by speech to the account of the being whose fault it is'. Reasoning that is immediately valid for the account of enjoyment: the one that is not is nonetheless inscribed in the act of saying as the one that is not appropriate, bringing it back once again to the starting square, that of phallic enjoyment which, for its part, feeds the act of saying until it is satiated.

There is not therefore just one enjoyment, to tell the truth, but it is ruled out that there are two of them. This right way puts a singular mark on the feminine enjoyment, an expression launched by Lacan, that he took up again on numerous occasions and which has known ever since a remarkable success, along a straight line from the biblical to each his own: to men phallic enjoyment (one would grant it also to little girls and to clitoral women) and to womanly women, feminine enjoyment. The trouble, on the Lacanian at least, is that 'if it existed [this feminine enjoyment], it should not be that one'. The reason why, let it be said in passing, not-man can be understood, while not (not man) does not present the same positivity.

However indefinite the act of saying may be, Lacan wants to affirm that something escapes it, that it can only be silent about, or exclude, or invoke, or reject, without ever for all of that managing to grasp it in the pincers of signification. The 'other enjoyment' strives to designate in this way, in its own way, the excess of the reference onto signification,[38] from the Fregean *Bedeutung* onto his *Sinn*. Because of this fact, one can say that it is central in the speaking being, but one can just as well say that it is nothing, no singular experience. It is without locus and accompanies phallic enjoyment as its shadow if it is true that the phallic makes this joining of the speaking subject to language and to the whole symbolic apparatus from which it depends, as much for its survival as for its existence, but from the rhetorical point of view, this other enjoyment is inscribed rather in the type of argumentation proper to the negative theologies. One can only invoke it in order to deny it since the reference is absent, but this absence is crucial for anyone who wants to appreciate the consistency of phallic enjoyment, the quality of its universality. We are soon going to see Lacan battle a foot at a time to establish a phallic function that is not reduced to a universality posed at first as such, in its classical extension. For the moment, it will be enough to record that this numbering of enjoyments resituates in its way the initial problem from which we started with the Biblical quotations: it is impossible to calmly count up to 2,[39] despite appearances, once it is a matter of establishing the difference of the genders on a sexual difference. This undeniable difference does not allow to be substantialised the terms that it opposes, to produce consistent genders; other hypotheses are required, most often silent ones, and without which the two remains out of reach.

Notes

1 New Revised Standard Version. In verse I, 27, this version has *humankind* in place of *man*.
2 The idea of a genealogical tree common to the species is deceptive here, because this tree is produced from top to bottom, from its unique summit towards its multiple bases, and only a reading coming after this mental construction may allow it to be believed that one could just as easily climb back from the multiple of the base towards the unicity of the summit. Now if we start from ourselves towards our ancestors, we unceasingly multiply the forbears. The lovers of genealogical trees know the problem. If from Adam to us the path may appear fairly direct, from us to Adam it is much riskier.
3 O. Boulnois, 'Un et un font un. Sexes, différences et union sexuelle au Moyen Âge, à partir des commentaires des Sentences', in *Ils seront deux en une seule chair, scénographie du couple humain dans le texte occidental*, edited by Pierre Legendre, Travaux du laboratoire européen pour l'étude de la filiation, Bruxelles, Emile Van Balberghe libraire, 2004, p. 115.
4 In a vast body of work, we chose for the present study: *La Querelle des universaux, de Platon à la fin du Moyen Âge*, Paris, Seuil, 1966, coll. '*Des travaux*', and the translation by Alain de Libera and A. Ph. Segonds of Porphyre *Isagogue*, Paris, Vrin, 1988. The very long introduction by A. de Libera is particularly rich.
5 This Roman, born at the end of the 5th century and dying in 524, was a senator, a consul, and then a counsellor of Theodoric, who exiled him and ended up having him executed. He was the translator of not only Porphyr's *Isagogue* but also of certain Aristotlean texts. The work which made him famous up to today is his *De consolatione philosophiae*.
6 Porphyr, *Isagogue*, op. cit., p. 1.
7 All the different translators are here already on the wheel. In order to translate the Greek, Tricot tries 'subsistent realities'. Confronted with the same term, A. de Libera chooses for his part the simple *exist* and cannot avoid two-and-a-half pages of very dense commentary to justify the choice of such a translation. Cf. Porphyr, *Isagogue*, op. cit., pp. 32–34.

8 E. Gilson, *La philosophie au Moyen Âge*, Paris, payot, 1942, pp. 142–143. Quoted by de Libera, *La Querelle. . . , op. cit.*, p. 39.
9 de Libera. *La Querelle, op. cit.*, p. 127.
10 Roscelin was born in the middle of the 11th century at Compiègne, studied at Soissons and at Reims, then taught in his native town, at Tours, at Loches (where he was Abelard's teacher), and finally at Besançon where he died around 1120.
11 I do not know how Roscelin organises this with Genesis II, 18–24. Does Eve belong to the human genus, or does she pass over to the incomplete human? Moreover, the argument is very cruel since at the time of these exchanges Abelard is himself no longer altogether complete.
12 This extreme conception of Roscelin of a semantic of reference could be very useful to anyone who would like to launch himself – this research still remains to be done – into a description of the semiotics of a certain Jacques Lacan. Even though always sketched out and never fully separated out, his conception of the sign makes so little of the signified that the referent often occupies in it a great place than one might image at first sight.
13 Quoted by de Libera, *La Querelle. . . , op. cit.*, p. 150.
14 Quoted by Alain Boulluec in his article 'From the unity of the couple to the union of Christ and the Church', in *Ils seront deux. . . , op. cit.*, p. 50.
15 Born at Toulouse, a Dominican and reader in theology, he was the bishop of Pamiers from 1326 until his death in 1347.
16 Quoted and translated by Gilbert Dahan in his article 'Genesis II, 23–24 in Christian exegesis', in *Ils seront deux. . . , op. cit.*, p. 102. Curiously, in his translation, G. Dahan drops the passage 'virago enim quasi acta de viro' . . . Pierre le Mangeur was, for his part, the chancellor of schools at Troyes from 1168 to 1178 and the author of a celebrated compilation of biblical history, known under the name of *Bible historiale.*
17 I am following here the presentation given by A. de Libera in his commentary on Boethius. *La Querelle. . . , op. cit.*, p. 130.
18 *Dictionnaire du Moyen Âge*, under the direction of C. Gauvard, A. de Libera and M. Zink, Paris, PUF, Quadrige, 2002, p. 2.
19 Hermaphrodism is not in question here as so far as it is conceived of either out of any class or belonging to both.
20 T. Laqueur, *Making Sex: Body and Gender from the Greek to Freud.* Cambridge, MA, Harvard University Press, 1992.
21 SE VII, p. 219.
22 SE XIX, p. 252.
23 SE VII, p. 219 n1.
24 SE XIX, 258.
25 S. Ferret, *Le Bateau de Thésée. Le problème de l'identité à travers le temps*, Paris, Éditions de Minuit, 1996.
26 A. Bourreau, *La Papesse Jeanne*, Paris, Flammarion, 1993.
27 Here, as elsewhere in the text, when each sex is considered as an essence, it is given a capital letter.
28 J. Lacan, *Écrits*, Paris, Le Seuil, 1966, pp. 725–734. In English, *Écrits*, translated by Bruce Fink, Norton, 2002, pp. 610–620. Announced as having been written 'two years before the Congress', this text is to be dated from 1958.
29 *Ibid.*, p. 732 (French) and p. 616 (English).
30 *Ibid.*, p. 735 (French) and p. 619 (English).
31 J. Lacan, *. . . or Worse*, 10 May 1972. For another translation of this rather obscure passage, see A. R. Price's translation, *. . . or Worse*, Polity, 2018, pp. 156–157.
32 *Le Grand Robert de la Langue francaise* respectively, tome I, p. 628, tome V; p. 1319.
33 J. Lacan, *Encore*, Paris, Le Seuil, 1975, p. 56.
34 '*Non decet*', says Lacan, arming himself with Latin to relaunch the equivocation between *convenir* (*decet*) and *dire* (*dicere*).
35 *Ibid.*, p. 57.

36 *Ibid.*, p. 56.

37 'I desire that what I will write should be taken only as a hypothesis, which is perhaps very far from the truth; but even if this were so, I believe I would have done a lot if all the things that are deduced from it are entirely in conformity with experience', R. Descartes, *Œuvres philosophiques*, tome III, Paris, Garnier-Flammarion, 1973, p. 247. This is exactly the kind of hypothesis that Newton declared that he did not want to forge in his physics.

38 In this way we can make sense of the specification contributed by Lacan in the session of 9 June 1971 of the seminar on *A Discourse That Might Not Be a Semblance*: 'much more rather I would insist on the fact that '*Die Bedeutung des Phallus*' is, in reality, a pleonasm. There is not in language any other *Bedeutung* than the phallus. Language in its function of existence, only connotes – I said connotes – in the final analysis the impossibility of symbolizing the sexual rapport among the beings that inhabit, that inhabit language, by reason of the fact that it is from this habitat that they have taken speech'.

39 Philip Larkin has given a short version of it: 'Thinking in terms of one / is easily done / one room, one bed, one chair / one person there, / makes perfect sense; one set / of wishes can be met / one coffin filled / but counting up to two / is harder to do / for one must be denied / before it's tried', *Collected Poems*, London, Faber & Faber, 1989, p. 108.

2

TOWARDS A CRITICAL READING OF THE FORMULAE OF SEXUATION

The provocative impression of Jacques Lacan's affirmation that 'there is no sexual *rapport*' continues to appear to many as a sort of brutal truth about sex, gaining authenticity by coming from a now-famous psychoanalyst. From this to imagining that it was simply his long experience as a practitioner that led him to this harsh truth about the nature of the relations men and women have (or not) with one another is an easy step to take. And besides, do not the apparently contradictory logical formulae which soon came to support and accompany in his teaching this paradoxical statement – produced at the end of the 1960s – place 'Man'[1] on one side and 'Woman' on the other? And so it is that for more than 30 years people have been satisfied to read these formulae as a modern set of magical spells in which, through a prodigious aggiornamento, biblical truth has finally found the place and the function of sexual difference in the vast Freudian setting, thanks to the somersaults of this entertainer Lacan. Nothing could be further from the truth. And what follows is intended to demonstrate this using the logical argumentation that Lacan developed over many years.

Carving into segments a teaching which spanned 27 years undoubtedly presents as many disadvantages as advantages, but to take such a long journey as a single block also generates an optical illusion that is fatal to any reading by reducing to a system what was, as it clearly proclaims from the beginning, a progressive elaboration, with its chaotic elements and its lightning flashes, its explorations and its avoidances. If from 1953 on, Lacan produced with his symbolic, imaginary, real triad an apt tool for undertaking a reading of the Freudian text which was not a professorial commentary, it was only at the beginning of the 1960s that he launched himself into innovations whose direct equivalents in Freud one will search for in vain. In saying this, I am not indicating either an epistemological or thematic break, and we can easily find such constructions in the course of the 1950s (the metonymical object, the foreclosure of the name of the father, etc.); much more rather a clear decision to introduce into the Freudian field what would deserve to be called (stealing the word from the mathematicians) 'ideal elements', the type of element that must be added to a set of already given elements in order to install in it, under certain conditions, a structure of a more powerful order. When in the course of his seminar on *Identification* (1961–1962) Lacan introduced his definition of the subject as *represented by a signifier for another signifier*, he was giving a place to such an entity which does not belong to the set that it regulates (the big Other, defined in this instance, as 'the treasury of signifiers'), but it was also this 'subject' which forced him to produce a quite different 'object' to that which up to then he had used under this same name of object.

Towards the object and its slight *rapport* to the one

He had already some presentiment of what he was then obliged to put forward as his own conception of what is understood by 'object':

> [T]he object o, as we are trying to define it, because it has become necessary for us now to have a proper definition of the object . . . to try to see how there is ordered, and at the same time differentiated what up to the present in our experience we have rightly or wrongly begun to articulate as being the object.[2]

But for him, this could only be done by right away rejecting the binary subject/object opposition, so true is it that his triplicity (ternarism), his way of counting three in everything, constrains him on this occasion. Here the quotations could be extremely numerous; let us be satisfied with the following:

> The whole notion of object relations is impossible to manage, impossible to comprehend, impossible even to use if we do not put into it as – I will not say a mediating element, because this would be to take a step that we have not yet taken together – a third element which is an element, in a word, of the phallus, which I am today putting centre stage with this schema: Mother/Phallus/Child.[3]

How was Lacan led to take more precautions here than his colleagues, who saw no difficulty in talking about an object in the common meaning of the term? By keeping before him his own conception of such an object, full of generous promise in its beginnings and thereafter extremely compromising if it proved to be the only one available: the specular image.

The problem is revelatory of Lacan's way of doing things and is worthwhile taking into account when we are proposing to read him: when he has put forward something that has some value in his eyes . . . he uses it until he abandons it or forgets it in favour of something else. In this sense, he is serious. He likes to make a series of what he is putting forward. He had thus produced, from his first steps in psychoanalysis, with his mirror stage and the most developed text that flowed from it,[4] a conception of the object on the exact model of the specular image: everything that will be brought forward in the future as 'object' will carry the trademark of this first object, this image in the mirror to which the child identifies and alienates itself in the same movement, by what Lacan called from then on the 'knot of imaginary servitude'. The expression is violent, but the idea determining it is no less so: the object, the *Gegenstand*, what confronts the subject, will never be anything other in its global make-up than a duplication of this specular image, with all the properties accruing to this image. This amounts to saying that the object will always be liable to a certain type of unity which Lacan qualifies at first as imaginary and which we know today corresponds to what he called much later 'unian':[5] an all-encompassing unity, which possesses its own circumscription,[6] which functions as a sack, very akin to a totalising unity and its vocation to gather together in an 'all' as many elements as you wish, in this case an infinity.

This conception did not fail to give rise to a difficulty: If the object and the other emerge from the same matrix, how can they be clearly differentiated? This question remains unresolved in *The Family*. Now it had to be dealt with successfully since the object of the drive, to limit ourselves to it, must be different from the small other. Two events, one positive and the other negative but both linked to a conception of unity, were going to lead to a way out.

During the seminar on *The Ethics of Psychoanalysis*, Lacan launched (for quite different reasons) into a commentary on the Freudian *Ding* as he found it in the *Project* (as opposed to *Sache*), which allowed him to glimpse what might be involved in a *non-narcissistic* (and thus nonspecular, not one?) object. Commenting on the Freudian distinction between 'ego-libido' and 'object-libido', he put forward the following:

> The object here, at this level, is introduced inasmuch as it is perpetually interchangeable with the love the subject has for his own image. . . . It is with this mirage-relation that the notion of object is introduced. This object is therefore not the same thing as the object aimed at on the horizon of the tendency. Between the object as structured by the narcissistic relation and *das Ding*, there is a difference . . .

In this term, with its distinguished philosophical and Freudian pedigree, Lacan found a first prop for thinking about an object that was not caught up in this 'knot of imaginary servitude' which, at least since 1938, the specular image had been for him. A path was opened up to think of the existence of a thing crucial in the subjective economy which, in Freud's own expression in the *Project*, escaped from the type of unity presented by any object worthy of the name. For most of those who took the risk of thinking anything whatsoever about the object in general, Leibniz's maxim according to which 'being and the one are equivalent' was, in effect, the rule, and one could not posit any object without by this very fact saying that it was 'one'. *Das Ding*, with its pretension of escaping from representation, by incarnating the part of judgement that cannot be articulated, opened up a path to enable there to be sustained the existence of an object which had broken its bonds with unity.

But what unity? During these same years, as he continued his commentary on Freud, Lacan gave a quite special role to the *einziger Zug* with which Freud had constructed hysterical identification to a 'singular' feature. In translating this expression by *unary trait* (*trait unaire*), Lacan chose to make of it one of the figures of the one, that in truth was indispensable for him, as he constructed his notion of 'signifier'. His supposed borrowings from Saussure in effect only offered him a differential concept of the signifier, each defined only as being different to all the others. With this notion of unary trait authorised by Freud, Lacan founded something different, a sort of atomism of the signifier which was to allow him to embody a notion of the letter that was entirely his own. We see it appearing clearly in his commentary on *The Purloined Letter* and still more in what followed the commentary that he gave when his *Écrits* appeared in 1966. If Lacan was able to affirm there with such assurance that a letter always arrives at its destination, it is not because there is any empirical evidence for this statement (contrary examples are only too obvious). It is an axiom which serves to define what a letter is: something indivisible at its very source because it stems from this unary trait, which is defined as possessing this type of unity which neither dissolves nor corrupts, a sort of irreducible unity of the basic element of the symbolic system.[7] Over and against a Derrida who was still to come, Lacan put in place a conception of a letter that could not be disseminated, foreign to any archive, to rats and to other accidents that could chip at it, spoil it, ruin it, and thus deviate it from its circuit as letter. No need here to lean towards a supposed 'nature' of what a letter truly is; we are here at the level of axiomatic statements; none is any truer than the other; we must choose the one whose consequences will assist what we want to appropriately support with it. Lacan holds that a letter should be defined by its circuit, and for that reason, he needs a letter which in its functioning possesses this 'unarity' which makes of it 'the localised structure of the signifier'. With it, Lacan henceforth possesses a type of unity which corresponds to his specular unity: inasmuch as the latter corresponds to an encompassing whole, the former validates the irreducible unity of the element. With two ones of this calibre under his belt, he can already go far, but he also realises . . . that neither is appropriate to give body and shape to an object which is not simply different but irreducible to the other, to this small other which, from its beginnings, provided a lodging place for all thought about the object.

Liable neither to imaginary and specular unity nor to unary: What then can be the *rapports* of the object still to come and the one? Thus posited, the question long in confinement in the progressive development of the seminars, could gradually hope to meet its answer . . . negative.

The object described as 'partial'

The seminar on *Transference* takes this problematic forward by proposing first of all, as regards this object in search of its new determinations, the notion of agalma. This Greek term, which Lacan said he had encountered and noted well before rediscovering it in the *Symposium*, designates, of course, a precious object, an ornament, an adornment, but what is most interesting to his eyes, is its brilliant aspect:

> What is at stake, is the brilliant meaning, the gallant meaning, because the word *gallant* comes from *galler* in old French.

Because of this insistence by Lacan on this 'brilliance' which the agalma is, a first shift of meaning is already at work: it is no longer just any object whatsoever that falls under the concept of agalma, it is much more rather a property of the object. Agalma, to put it in Aristotelian terms, is not so much a being as an accident, less a substantive than an adjective. And nevertheless, Lacan brings it forward and clearly considers it as an object, without for a single instant making of it a universal in the medieval mode. It is not a matter, in effect, of considering the agalma as 'the' brilliant, a brilliant to which one would lend an existence outside the objects on which it is brought to bear. It is an object . . . which has not the full and stable being that one usually expects of an object, which one believes in advance to be everything at once: a substantive in language, perduring in space and time, endowed with a being that makes it participate in a natural ontology and so forth. The agalma for its part is presented right away as out of synch as compared to this plenitude.

What is more is, having barely been put forward in this way, we see this object energetically attached to the analytic notion of 'part-object' but in a very curious way! Following the same thread as this idea of 'gallant', Lacan continues, immediately after the previous quotation:

> It is indeed, it must be said what we analysts have discovered under the name of part object. This function of part object is one of the greatest discoveries of analytic investigation.[8]

This long and learned development on the term *agalma* ends then with a sudden sidestep: Lacan had been talking about the 'part-object'! But what is this yoke which is declared to be 'one of the greatest discoveries of analytic investigation'? To understand the manoeuvre we have to forget what we believe we know so well about this part object . . . due to the later work of a certain Jacques Lacan.

On 1 February 1961, the term *part-object* had a familiar resonance in the ears of the listeners only because of a certain Melanie Klein, who had promoted it for more than 20 years. Then it was spoken about, above all, in English as 'part-object'. And for her, this part-object had nothing to do with the agalma that Lacan is in the process of sketching out before his listeners. Here is a first complication that it is important to sort out.

The false Freudian trail

The word *partial* has undoubtedly the dignity of coming from Freud. Since the *Three Essays on the Theory of Sexuality* Freud had used it right through his description of the workings of the drive. The problem is that he never uses it at the level of the object of the drive, which is always said to be 'indifferent' (*quelconque*) and never 'partial'. What is described as partial are the 'sources' of the drives, in the very precise sense that with the second pubertal instinctual surge, these sources (oral, anal) are going to have to converge towards the 'primacy of the genital'. This later convergence is what alone makes them 'partial' during the time of infantile sexuality, this partiality remaining one of the constant components of these drives, even once there has been established (very problematically, seen from today) this genital convergence.

The first notch in this construction comes from Karl Abraham who towards the end of his long text *A Short Study of the Development of the Libido, Viewed in the Light of Mental Disorders* (1924), in the chapter titled 'Origins and Growth of Object-Love',[9] comes to forge the expression 'partial love of the object', starting from which Melanie Klein is going to invent something quite different: her part-object.

This is not the place to enter into the complex relations maintained in this author between her part-objects (which, at the start, closely copy the Freudian oral and anal sources but multiply very quickly) and the 'total object' which certainly appears during the depressive phase but is already found to operate in the previous schizo-paranoiac phase.[10] It would be well on the contrary to clearly appreciate against whom the irony that Lacan immediately deploys regarding this subject is directed:

> We ourselves have also effaced, as far as we could, what is meant by the partial object; namely, that our first effort was to interpret what had been a marvelous discovery, namely, this fundamentally partial aspect of the object in so far as it is the pivot, centre, key of human desire, this would have been worth dwelling on for a moment. . . . But no, not at all! It was directed towards a dialectic of totalisation, namely, the only one worthy of us, the flat object, the round object, the total object, the spherical object without feet or paws, the whole of the other, the perfect genital object at which, as everyone knows, our love irresistibly comes to term.[11]

The target here is not so much Melanie Klein as the French analysts whom Lacan has so much against at this time, in general, those who had just published *La Psychanalyse aujourd'hui* (*Psychoanalysis Today*), in first place, Maurice Bouvet. In his attack against the authors who are inventing, in effect, a genital object (that Freud himself had not supported), Lacan passes off as a discovery of Freud's something that is nothing other than an invention of his own: the partial object with a totally unexpected meaning, an object which does not come from any totality, does not belong nor is not destined to any and for which the Greek term of *agalma* comes to offer its shelter, in direct succession to the metonymical object, half-object/half-phallus/half-signifier, already squeezed between what in the signified will remain beyond signification, without for all that connecting up with the worldly opacity of the linguistic referent.[12]

This boisterous irony designates, just by itself, what is at stake in this partial, that Lacan presents as the most precious asset of the Freudian analytic tradition, even though no one before him had ever dreamt of producing, under the name of 'object', a 'partial' which was not part of any whole, never called to integrate any 'whole' whatsoever. From 1 February 1961 on, we can consider that the o-object, present for almost five years in the seminars, has broken its ties with the small other (it is said to be 'non-specular'), and has acquired the determination that leads it towards a consistency that is quite its own: this 'partial' whose status remains to be assured. This is no slight matter, and begins with a sort of brawl with Kant himself.

The Kantian *nihil negativum*

That Lacan was at that time clearly conscious of the new epistemological implications of his theoretical exigencies can be divined by perusing the whole of the seminar that follows *Transference*, namely, *Identification*. On 28 February 1962 for example he states:

> It is quite clear in any case that there is no room for admitting as tenable Kant's transcendental aesthetics, despite what I called the unsurpassable character of the service he performs for us in his critique, and I hope to make this felt by what I am going to show is to be substituted for it.

What then is the introductory point at which Lacan appeals to Kant? It is so unclear that there is no other recourse than to follow his progress step by step. He found himself that day talking about life drive/death drive and about Freud's necessity to sustain his idea of the life drive by that of narcissism – to the point of closely studying the question of pain in *On Narcissism: An Introduction*. He then recalls – why the devil, what had gotten under his skin? – that during a casual conversation a little earlier, he had pointed out to his listener that the experience of one pain blots out that of another, in short, that it is difficult to suffer two pains at the same time. He continues:

> One dominates, makes you forget the other, as if the libidinal investment on your own body shows itself to be subject to the same law of partiality that motivates the relation to the world of objects of desire.

So here then there are collected together like the umbrella and the sewing machine on the dissecting table, the partiality of the object – a quite recent invention as we have seen – and the operation of the primary processes (libidinal cathexis) in its relationship to the body, when Lacan unceremoniously declares:

> And here is where, as I might say, the reference to, the analogy with Kant's investigation is going to be of use to us.

Surprisingly, Lacan first sets about a kind of crude disqualification of Kantian aesthetics. 'It is absolutely not tenable', he says, 'for the simple reason that for him [Kant] it is fundamentally supported by a mathematical argumentation that stems from what one can call '*L'époque géométrisante de la mathématique*' (the geometricising epoch of mathematics'.[13]

This word *géométrisant* just by itself announces something: up to Cantor/Dedekind, the only available continuity was geometrical continuity. It was by this fact the only one suitable for representing irrational numbers, the numbers that do not result from any *rapport* of numbers, such as $\sqrt{2}$ so that this number and all its peers belonged indeed to the 'geometricising epoch of mathematics'. Once Cantor and Dedekind, each in his own way, founded numerical continuity, the question is presented quite differently, and this is how Lacan intends to treat it, from his first attack on Kant.

In this context, Lacan remains some pages of Kant's *Critique of Pure Reason*, namely the end of the chapter 'On Amphibology of Concepts of Reflection', where Kant takes care to line up four different nothings. Lacan ironises about the example that Kant gives to illustrate the last instance of his table of nothings, the *leer Gegenstand ohne Begriff*, namely a rectilinear figure which would only have two sides. And the epicycloids, asks Lacan? Is it not in direct contradiction with such a definition and has been known since Pascal! The rest of this session remains woolly in its relationship to the Kantian text, Lacan insisting on a certain *ens privativum*, which is enough to indicate some vacillation since Kant never employs such an expression.

In his table of four nothings that closes the 'Note to the Amphibology of Concepts of Reflection',[14] Kant aligns in effect in this order *ens rationis* (the empty concept without an object, the banal 'nothing'), *ens imaginarium* (the empty intuition without an object, like time or space, the simple forms of intuition that have no right to the name of 'object'), the *nihil privativum* (the negation of something, therefore the concept of the lack of the object, like cold or shadow), and finally the *nihil negativum*, the *leer Gegenstand ohne Begriff*, the empty object without a concept that Lacan had almost disqualified, in his previous and imprecise Kantian vocabulary. The tone changes in the following session, 28 March 1962:

> Every time we analysts have to deal with this *rapport* of the subject to the nothing, we regularly slip between two slopes: the common slope that tends

> towards a nothing of destruction . . . and the other which is the nihilisation that could be assimilated to Hegelian negativity.

He continues in a Kantian vocabulary that this time is much more rigorous since he spells out then, in order, Kant's four nothings:

> The nothing that I am trying to get to hold together for you at this initial moment in the establishment of the subject is something else. The subject introduces the nothing as such and this nothing is to be distinguished from any classical negativity [this is the Kantian '*ens rationis*'], from any imaginary being which is that of a being whose existence is impossible [this is the Kantian '*ens imaginarium*'], the famous centaur which brings the logicians, indeed the metaphysicians to a halt at the beginning of their path towards science, which is not either the *ens privativum* [instead of '*nihil privativum*', here Lacan repeats his slip from the previous session], which is properly speaking what Kant in the definition of his four nothings, admirably called the *nihil negativum*, namely, to use his own terms: *leer Gegenstand ohne Begriff*, an empty object, but let us add, without concept, without any grip on it being possible.[15]

In the space of a month, Kant has gone from what is highlighted as a zero in mathematics to an 'admirable invention' in connection with the same thing, this 'nothing', this 'empty object without a concept' which interests Lacan in his completely new approach to 'partiality' because it offers a refuge for an object which, by definition, escapes from the unity of the concept, from this minimal grasp which puts into rapport anything whatsoever with the one, when we try to think about it. What is at stake then is indeed to combat the Kant of the transcendental aesthetics but not without borrowing from him in passing what allows there to be sustained the term *object* by preventatively disengaging it from any *rapport* to the one, under the privative form of an absence of concept.

This strange recourse by Lacan to one of the most eccentric points of the great Kantian corpus is too often neglected on the pretext that he does not come back to it once he had gone past the quotations that we have just read; but this is to condemn oneself to not understanding what is at stake for him vis-à-vis unity in the course of the constitution of his partial object, from its very first steps. This object must not pass either under the Caudine Forks of specular unity or under those of the unary; the too-welcoming inn of the concept must therefore be immediately withdrawn from it because it would bring it back, silently, under the auspices of the most classical unity. But why does Lacan on several occasions and with a gap of more than a month, while very obviously he has reread the Kantian text very carefully, make this same slip which makes him invent an *ens privativum*?

Lacan/Freud: the privative object

With such an expression, undeniably his own, he is holding then, against Kant, that there is here a being and not a nothing, even though the *Critique of Pure Reason* presents it straight out as a nothing coming from a lack:

> Reality is *some thing*, negation is *nothing*, namely, a concept of the lack of the object, like shadow or cold (*nihil privativum*).[16]

The matter is clarified if one considers that this lack of object constitutes a quasi-definition of the Freudian object, which will never be anything other than the shadow carried over from the mythical object of the first satisfaction. This Freudian object takes on, in the eyes of Lacan, the status of lost object (and phallic lack is its flagship) because Freud thinks of his object under the category of *nihil privativum*, of the 'object empty of a concept', as Kant also puts it, understanding, of course, here a positive concept, referring to a classical object, which, in this instance, is missing. Negation in this case has impacted on the positive object, and there results this *nihil privativum*, but this operation itself leaves intact the category of object and its ineradicable *rapport* to the one.

Here then I am making the hypothesis that the repeated slip by Lacan on this point comes from the fact that he reads 'Freud' in the word *lack* present in Kant and fabricates by this fact this curious *ens privativum*, this object of privation.[17] Now the nothing that he is trying to promote is differentiated from the 'Freudian lack' as well as from 'Hegelian negativity' that we have seen him denounce as being both foreign to his purposes.[18] In short, he sees himself as being alone on the side of the *nihil*; he relegates the others (Freud, Hegel, Bouvet, and company), each in his own way, to the side of being, of the *ens*, at the very least to a simple syntactic negation of being, while he is striving to sustain the paradoxical existence of a 'nothing' cleansed of any essence. Here starts the matter of the 'non-rapport'.

Towards non-*rapport*

Pressing on now to get to what pushed Lacan, thanks to an audacious conception of non-*rapport*, to radicalise the wager he had inaugurated at the beginning of the 1960s, by this innovation of an unprecedented partial, I will leave here in relative shadow two dimensions which are the object of numerous sessions of the seminar between 1961 and 1967: the one that, through the Fibonacci series, tries to tie together the *rapports* of the 0-object and numerical unity and the other which, playing on topology, offers him a definition of specularity – the inversion of the orientation of a surface in its specular image – which allows there to be envisaged the non-specularity of this very 0-object otherwise than in the style of the vampire (known for not having an image in the mirror).

A serious reading of these two working axes of Lacan in the 1960s would nevertheless not be superfluous. It would allow there to be better isolated the conditions encountered by Lacan in the establishing of the 0-object as he knew he needed it and that no other tradition, either philosophical or mathematical, offered to him on a plate. I content myself here with a remark relative to the Fibonacci series.

This will, in effect, allow Lacan to indicate, thanks to a daring metaphor, the *rapport* between signifier and 0-object. The law of composition of the series is expressed in modern terms:

$$U_n = U_{n-1} + U_{n-2},$$

the two first terms being equal to unity. There is thus produced the following numerical series:

1, 1, 2, 3, 5, 8, 13, 21, 34, 55, 89, 144, 233, 377, 610, 987, 1597, 2584, etc.

The arithmetical reason of this progression, U_{n-1}/U_n proves to be equal to 0.61803989 . . . , in other words, the golden number encountered by Euclid in his division of the segment unity (which he calls 'the whole'!) into 'mean and extreme reason'. Now this number – that Lacan is quick to name 'a' – presents astonishing properties, among others it is the same whether it divides the unity or is added to it: $1/a = 1 + a$. One can certainly not say that it does not entertain any *rapport* with unity – and in this sense, it is incorrect to take over the 0-object (l'objet [a]) under this aspect – but at least it is the only one to propose such a bizarre relation with the one. There is that already. But there is more, and Lacan echoes it, rather tardily, at a moment when he is ready to abandon this series and its astonishing properties. On 11 June 1969, towards the end of the seminar *From an Other to the Other*, he acknowledges to his listeners:

> If I am talking to you about the Fibonacci series, it is because of the following. That in the measure that the figures that represent it increase, the relationship U_{n-1}/U_n is more and more close, more and more rigorously strictly equal to what we have called, and not by chance although in another context, by the same sign that we designate the 0-object. This little irrational o, equal to $\frac{1+\sqrt{5}}{2}$, is something that is perfectly stabilized as a *rapport* in the measure that there is generated the representation of the subject by a numerical signifier with regard to another numerical signifier.

This was, in effect, where he wanted to get to: the Fibonacci series offers us the elegant metaphor of a signifying series which is found to approximate always better in its development to the same value, which will never belong to the series, and which maintains with unity the strange *rapports* that we have just seen. In short, the more the signifying series is extended, the better there is circumscribed, without ever touching it, what is at stake in the 0-object, already defined also as 'object cause of desire' (to say nothing here about its other subjective uses), a whole program for a psychoanalyst set on giving to his listeners a certain conception of analytic treatment, since the idea of an intrinsic end to the transferential adventure is already inscribed in such a metaphor.

If it articulates in a (little too) happy way signifying production and the constant escape of this 0-object which has taken over from the metonymical object, the Fibonacci series remain powerless to generate any non-rapport to the one which would express the value that Lacan intends to give to his 'partial'. In this year of 1969, this series invoked here and there for almost 10 years had been squeezed dry and must hand over to something else for there to be said what remained silent with it.

I will be still more allusive about the topological efforts of Lacan who, being helped by one of the properties of the specular image (the inversion of left/right relationships), is going to name as 'non-specular' the surfaces, well known by mathematicians at that time under the name of 'non-orientable' surfaces, which do not possess this reflexive property of inverting orientation: the Moebius strip, the Klein bottle, and the cross-cap are thus going to be unfurled in the seminars of the 1960s to try to give a place to everything which, in analytic practice and the conception of the treatment, escapes from the tentacular grasp of the specular image.

Whatever may be the intrinsic merits of these numerical and topological resources, I start from the idea that none of them was able to offer to Lacan the material to sustain the intuition guiding him since, at least, the seminar *On Transference* and its promotion of an unprecedented partial: that the object as we must conceive of it following the thread of Freudian experience was to be excluded from any rapport to the one, required much more than the discovery of a knowledge that was already there, ready to welcome such a thing.

This intuition of a partial ungraspable in the pincers of unity has for Lacan mathematical roots,[19] but it has also on its side a poetic and political force that it would be a pity to ignore, because this is where it derives the essential of its force, well before finding the slightest clinical relevance. Unity possesses of course at least two aspects (see Parmenides where Plato enumerates them, among others), those that Lacan for his part distinguishes as 'unary' and 'unian'. But here the partial that is being profiled is said to escape both from the one and the other: its obstinate quality of object allows it – we do not really know how – not to fall under any of these 'ones'. It presents itself then as a perfect cartoon character, a mongrel Pinocchio: liberated with its first steps from any slavery to a concept, rebellious to the 'knot of imaginary servitude' of the specular image, and immediately linked to the drive and to desire, it is ready to gambol to left and to right and in this very way to accomplish for its Geppetto, its inventor, multiple and varied tasks. Except that, like all these extravagant little characters, it has its own requirements: it must be nourished in non-rapport, since its destiny obliges it not to enter into rapport with the one (which would bring it back to the concept, like the Prodigal Son), hence the necessity of writing such a thing; otherwise, Lacan knew that he would find himself in a poetic-mystical position that, certainly he did not despise but in which he was not decently allowed to establish himself, given his practical credos, and his concern for rationality.

The coming of the formulae of sexuation

Here I am not going to carry out the scrupulous textual tracking that would lead us from a first (and very risky) 'There is no sexual act' (since *The Logic of Phantasy*) to 'There is no sexual *rapport*' which is spread throughout *Of a Discourse That Might Not Be a Semblance* and . . . *or Worse*. I content myself with marking some key moments in this progress that will culminate in the formulae called 'of sexuation', because it is they who try to write what is involved in the sexual non-rapport. The business begins with *Of a Discourse That Might Not Be a Semblance*, particularly in the session of 17 February 1971.

It is not the first time that Lacan articulates the expression according to which 'there is no sexual *rapport* in the speaking being', but that day, he is going to go further into detail of the considerations that produce such a statement. He invokes the signs used by modern biology to designate the masculine and the feminine, then the Chinese Yin and Yang, and still other couples that all aspire to express a form of sexual bi-partition. But what objects to such a binary classification, what ensures that it is 'untenable to remain in any way at this duality as sufficient', is once again the function described as the phallus, which always acts as a hindrance to counting on the base of two:

> [T]his function of the phallus renders henceforth untenable this sexual bipolarity, and untenable in a way that literally volatilizes what is involved in terms of what can be written about this rapport.[20]

If from 1956 on, this phallus sufficed, qua 'third element which is an element' (cf. the earlier discussion) to raise an objection to the subject/object couple, it is no longer under the heading of 'element' that it intervenes here but as 'function of the phallus' and soon the 'phallic function' (*fonction phallique*). This feminising and this adjectiving are heavy with consequences, for we no longer are dealing with an object (symbolic, mythical) but indeed with a rapport since a function, in the mathematical or logical vocabulary that Lacan is so fond of (he borrows this 'function' especially from Frege), is nothing other than a putting into rapport of elements belonging to two disjoined series. The 'phallic function' is then, in principle and by definition, the writing of a rapport. That is even all it is. Nevertheless, the two series that Lacan links or distinguishes by this function of the phallus are in no case men and women but speaking beings, on one hand, and enjoyment, on the other. This phallic function henceforth names the rapport of each speaking being, each *parlêtre*, to enjoyment. Lacan can henceforth add that the phallus understood in this way 'in no way designates the organ described as the penis with its physiology'.

'All the women'

As often when he introduces something new, Lacan likes to recall that he had already said it a long time ago, hence a reminder of 'The Direction of the Treatment and the Principles of its Power', a text in which he opposed, on the exact point of the phallus, in effect, the fact of 'being' it (reserved rather for women in this context) and that of 'having' it, reserved rather for men (but in order to have it, one must again accept not being it – cf. a certain type of impotence – and in order to be it again, one must accept not having it – cf. a certain mode of frigidity). What is now announced appears nevertheless more promising in the measure that Lacan talks here about a 'substitution for the sexual rapport of what is called the sexual law'. Now what do we see appearing in the minutes that follow this 'substitution'? Nothing other than the presentation of the universal and particular, affirmative and negative propositions given by Peirce (and presented by Lacan himself during the seminar on *Identification* almost 10 years previous), which are now going to be used by him to write this 'sexual law', which aspires to articulate the rapport of each sex to enjoyment – to make then of the phallic function what will allow him to differentiate man and woman, to construct this difference, and thus to cease holding it as a primary (biblical) given on which all the rest could be constructed. This recourse to logic is preceded by a rapid but crucial mention of *Totem and Taboo*:

> The maintaining, the maintaining in analytic discourse of this residual myth that is called the Oedipus complex, God knows why, which is in fact that of *Totem and Taboo*, in which there is inscribed this myth that is entirely invented by Freud, of the primordial father in so far as he enjoys all the women, it is all the same here that we ought to question a little further from the point of view of logic and of writing, what it means. It is a long time since I introduced here the schema of Peirce.[21]

Here we have pronounced, as coming from the Freud of *Totem and Taboo* who can do nothing about it,[22] an 'all the women' which is going to reveal itself to be crucial in the operations that follow inasmuch as Lacan intends to deny it energetically and to sustain that nothing of the kind exists. He can subsequently hook this assertion onto something or other about feminine enjoyment, but the starting point is Freudian: it is Jacques Lacan's way of writing the Oedipal myth. 'All the women': not there. Starting from there, he is going to be able to deploy his questioning vis-à-vis the standing of the universal:

> What the myth of the enjoyment of all the women designates, is that there are not all the women. *There is no universal of the woman*. Here is what is posed by a questioning of the phallus, and not of sexual rapport, as regards what is involved in the enjoyment it constitutes, because I said that it was feminine enjoyment. It is starting from these statements that a certain number of questions can be radically displaced.[23]

A great trumpet blast, but we are still far from seeing clearly here. The immediately following passage, which deals with the fact that truth and falsity are only treatable in the dimension of the written, insists on the same point without making it any more convincing. All that we have for the moment is on the side described as 'man', a universal that one can describe as classical and on the other, on the side of 'woman', because of this very partial mention, for the moment, of *Totem and Taboo*, the negation of another universal, the declaration, for the moment strange, of its inexistence.[24]

First attempts

It is then, towards the end of the following session, that of 17 March 1971, that Lacan takes up again what he had brought from Peirce, about the phallus qua rapport to enjoyment, marked by the letter Φ, and the 'quantors' (or quantifiers) in order to begin to write all of that with the literal equipment of modern – let us say, post-Fregean – logic:

> the universal affirmative: $\forall x.\Phi x$ (for any x, phi of x)
> the particular affirmative: $\exists x.\Phi x$ (there exists an x such that phi of x)

Having got to the universal negative (e), the first difficulty;

> $\forall x.\overline{\Phi x}$ I want to express that this is a negative. How can I do so? I am struck by the fact that it has never been really articulated the way I am going to do it. What you have to do is to put a bar of negation above the Φx and not at all, as is usually done above both ($\overline{\forall x.\Phi x}$). And here, it is on the $\exists x$ that you have to put the bar ($\overline{\exists x}.\Phi x$, particular negative).

The reader not really accustomed to reading Lacan in a critical way is confronted here with a serious problem of attribution. This non-classical way of using the sign of negation by putting it, not on the totality of the proposition but only on each composant, is no longer that original at that time, even if Lacan presents it as one of his 'invention'. The fact is that he is going to give them new terms, *forclusion* (foreclosure) and *discordance* (discordance) borrowed from the French grammarians Damourette and Pichon. To get convinced of that is rather easy: it is enough to read the page 25 of Robert Blanché's book *Les Structures intellectuelles*,[25] where the author produces, from the universal affirmative (*universally p*) the three other propositions of the logical square, distinguishing a 'strong' negation that falls only on the function and gives the universal negative (*universally non-p*) and a 'weak' negation that falls only on the quantifier to give the particular negative (*non-universally p*), which already is the 'pas-tout' Lacan is looking for ($\overline{\forall x}.\Phi x$). That goes on to the particular affirmative, of course, which is consequently written *non-universally non-p* (since it has to contradict the universal negative [*universally non-p*], as we will see more in detail studying the functioning of the logical squares), which is what we encounter, with a nuance of writing,[26] in Lacan's formula: $\exists x.\overline{\Phi x}$. I would readily add that

Blanché could not be ignored by Lacan at that time since he is present in the issue n°10 of *Les Cahiers pour l'analyse*, in a paper[27] into which this system of double negation is clearly put forward.

Independent of that, this 17 March 1971, in his first attempt to write the four places of the logical square that are respectively the universal positive and negative and their corresponding particulars, Lacan then writes the series:

$$\forall x \Phi x \text{ (a) } \exists x.\Phi x \text{ (i); } \forall x.\overline{\Phi x} \text{ (e); } \overline{\exists x}.\Phi x \text{ (o).}$$ [28]

It is with the negation of the universal that Lacan says he has invented what he almost immediately names the 'non-value of the universal negative' (we know that he has already in his mind 'there is no all women'), a non-value from which he draws by way of a final commentary, this assertion: 'it is here [with the universal negative as he understands it], that there functions an essential cut, well then it is even around this that there is articulated what is involved in the sexual rapport'.

We note right away – we who know what the Lacan of 17 March 1971 does not yet know that the bar of negation does not fall on that day on the quantifier to produce the famous 'not-all' (written $\overline{\forall x}.\Phi x$, that will come only on 19 May), but only on the function itself, involving henceforth this $\forall x.\overline{\Phi x}$ whose existence will be short.[29] The particular negative is constructed with the other half of the negation, that falls on the existential quantifier producing a $\overline{\exists x}.\Phi x$ not very interesting, that will explicitly disappear very soon. Despite this distinction between two negations, it is clear that Lacan is still looking for, on this 17 March, how to write as well the universal negative as its particular, in the sense he tries to establish relatively to the sexual rapport. This writing is nevertheless not classical since it denies not the entirety of the universal affirmation (to be written $\overline{\forall x.\Phi x}$) but says that for any x, it must be denied that Φx is the case.

Here there is situated already the uncoupling which, on this 17 March, still remains to be correctly written. At this point, Lacan remembers Peirce, even as he is proposing to rewrite Aristotle (but we will soon see what in Aristotle) with the function and the quantification invented by Frege. At that moment, he again makes a big deal of what he says he owes to this same Peirce, namely that the absence of any stroke (the universal negative) confirms the universal affirmative: any and every stroke is vertical.[30] He omits, remarkably, noting that the absence of any stroke does not verify only the universal affirmative but anything and everything since, as the mathematicians know, if there is no x, if $x \in \varnothing$, x verifies any property whatsoever. The point that Lacan wants to underline, on the contrary, is that the quantifier of the universal, $\forall$, does not involve any necessity as regards existence, over and against the quantifier rightly described as 'existential', $\exists$, which for its part implies the existence of what he will soon name elsewhere in his teaching as the 'at-least-one' (*au-moins-un*), indeed *l'hommoinzun*.

∀ and the question of belonging

So then when we say (but more again when we write) 'for any man', this 'any man' which does not imply any existence, shows a quite singular status since we are going to predicate certain things about this being. Where is it? What is it? 'When it is subject', says Lacan on 19 May 1971, 'it implies a function of the universal which only gives it as support very specifically its symbolic status'. Here then is posited the question of belonging, in so far as it is not enough to settle the question of existence.

The operator 'for any' (∀) only has meaning in effect by referring the letter that follows it to an individual by which it is then written that it 'belongs' to a determined set. It is not 'indifferent' in itself, as Frege had already pointed out;[31] it results from any designation whatsoever in the set to which it belongs, which poses in a decisive way the question of the set in question. To employ this quantifier, is *ipso facto* to make the hypothesis that this set – that Frege called the 'range of values' of the variable – well and truly exists and that it is therefore permitted to take from it one element or another provided one has the right pincers (the right function, the one it satisfies). By showing that such sets do not always exist (to the great surprise of Frege), Bertrand Russell raised in a decisive way the question of paradoxes,[32] and Hilbert himself, in the program that he subsequently elaborated to settle the question of the foundations of mathematics, had taken the initial decision to get rid of this quantifier and the domain that it silently covers since both, in their way, reintroduced the question of the infinite by the fact of the belonging of the element thus isolated to an infinite set.[33]

I have tried to show that the subjective note of the universal stems, for each one, from the mystery of his strange assent to the idea that one day he will die.[34] On one hand, narcissism has a fundamental incapacity to envisage such a thing, and on the other, there is an unqualified certainty. If, instead of being left in the dark by such a split, we approach the certitude at stake in this instance, we see that the 'all' that it is a question of joining up with in recognising the absolute absence of exception to this rule of the species, is equivalent to eliminating oneself mentally from belonging to the order of the living and thus *a fortiori* from the species that belongs to it. 'All men are mortal' only has meaning from the moment when one who says 'I' accepts belonging to this set which says, for his part, in his quasi definition, that he is ridding himself of himself since to belong to it amounts to accepting to abstract himself from it. 'All men', far from empirically collecting the living in order to assemble them into an 'all' into which one would only have to go and be inscribed, is only obtained by liquidating the narcissistic exception that I am in the question of this 'all'. Induction here only succeeds in the measure that it manages to swallow up its inductor, and every man consents, from his deliberate start in this matter to his full and entire belonging to the species being, *in his essence*, a thought event by which he absents himself in advance from the all to which he aspires to belong. I only arrive as 'any man' in the measure that this 'any man' that I am, that I want to be, is capable of drawing a line over his existence while he is alive. The universal is a hard conquest; nonetheless, it comes with an amazing easiness.

On 19 May 1971, Lacan, in order to make himself understood on this point, does not launch himself into such aporias. He uses the roots of second degree equations, which do not all belong to real numbers (since some, the roots of negative numbers, belong to imaginary numbers), in order to make it understood that one can meet cases in which the particular affirmative and the particular negative, far from excluding one another, are in agreement (we will soon see the whole importance of this nuance). It nevertheless remains that, in every case, when we write that any element whatsoever 'belongs' to a determined set, we posit such a set as existing. No $\forall$ without the set that it is supposed to cover. And if no set . . .

Starting from the negation brought to bear on 'all women', Lacan concludes to the inexistence of 'The' woman as a strictly symbolic entity, and by that alone, there vanishes the possibility of writing a rapport between an entity possessing a set of values to be covered (men) and another which does not possess such a 'range of Fregean values' (women). Because there is no set of all women (in a way that is basically homogenous to the fact that there is 'no set of all the sets that do not belong to themselves'), there cannot be 'any woman' (any one at all insofar as she is supposed to belong to the set 'Women'), and so then there is no 'The' woman. QED (all of this under the starting condition – which for its part is enigmatic – that 'there is no all women').

The migration of negation: discordance and foreclosure

From this there derives the importance of the operator of negation in Lacan's eyes, to the point that he does not manage all that quickly to situate it correctly with regard to his own requirements. By first denying the function and not the quantifier (March 1971), he was still searching, as he acknowledges in all simplicity on 19 May 1971, qualifying as 'ineptitude' his previous writing of the universal negative under the form $\forall x.\overline{\Phi x}$:

> I slipped quite naturally, by trusting the memory of what it is a matter of rearticulating, I slipped over to writing it, namely, that the function, with its little bar above, symbolised something completely inept with respect to what I had effectively to say. You have perhaps noticed that, it never entered my head, at least up to the present, nor yours either, to think that the bar of negation perhaps had something to do, to say, not in the right-hand column but in the left. Let us try, what advantage can we draw from it?

And here then is a negation that falls no longer on a proposition, namely on a quantified function, but sometimes on a quantifier (producing the particular negative), sometimes on the function (producing the universal negative), in a way that is inverted as compared to the first formulae of 17 March. Lacan (following here

Robert Blanché or his own inspiration) writes then his two particulars (negative on left, affirmative on right):

$\overline{\forall x}.\Phi x$ and $\exists x.\overline{\Phi x}$

> There is a world, Lacan continues, between the two negations, the one which ensures that I do not write it, that I exclude it, and, as someone who was a rather subtle grammarian formerly expressed it, it is *forclusive.* The function will not be written. *I want to know nothing about it.* The other is *discordant.*

We might hesitate a little as regards knowing how to distribute the adjectives, but on 8 December 1971, right at the beginning of . . . *or Worse,* Lacan could not be clearer: 'Our not-all is discordance'. How understand these grammarian details in such a setting?

Rather simply, the discordant, as its name indicates rather well, and for once Damourette and Pichon do not have recourse to their learned farrago, is what introduces discord, discordance, disagreement. It is a way not yet of denying (this will be the work of foreclosure) but to mark a separation, a distance introduced in French by the first sign of negation 'ne'. Damourette and Pichon read its finest and most expressive nuance in the occasional use of this *ne* after the expression *avant que* (before) a turn of phrase, they say, that was gaining ground in the French of their time:

> Il sera parti avant que tu arrives; Il sera parti avant que tu n'arrives

[Both translated in English as 'He will be gone before you come']

The first use signals the brute fact of coming; the second reinforces the subjunctive summoned in French by the expression *avant que,* thus underlining the *possibility* of the fact, more than the fact itself.

Foreclosure, for its part, comes in these indispensable complements of negation, such as *pas, rien, jamais, aucun, personne, plus, guère, mie, goutte* (*no, nothing, never, any, no one, anymore, scarcely, at all, anything*), and so on. They apply, Damourette and Pichon continue, 'to facts that the speaker does not envisage as forming part of reality'.[35] In strong opposition then to the discordant which for its part envisages very well that what it is brought to bear on forms part of reality while introducing into it decisive nuances: *pastout* (not-all) does not say that there is nothing but that what there is does not give form to any whole.

These grammatical details are not enough, to my way of thinking, to give all its clarity to what Lacan then undertakes in order to subvert the meaning and the import of the universal negative. They nevertheless allow it to be seen right away that it is no longer a matter of producing a couple in opposition of the true/false type but that the universal affirmative and the universal negative henceforth maintain a sort of commerce, just as, in the same way, *discordance* and *foreclosure* are at the basis of the riches of negation in French inasmuch as they situate different postures in the rejection and the exclusion of an action, posited in another way in the proposition.

We thus progress with Lacan, through what he calls (8 December 1971) 'two quite different forms of negation', from a stated distance with regard to a function (through a 'weak' negation of the quantifier, from what there is discordance) to his entire rejection, his 'foreclosure' through the negation of the function, reinforced by the fact that there does indeed exist one who sustains this extreme of negation, which is henceforth brought to bear, no longer on the proposition (which would then be written $\overline{\exists x.\Phi x}$) but on the function: $\exists x.\overline{\Phi x}$.

On 3 March 1972 in the course of *The Knowledge of the Psychoanalyst*, Lacan again gives some details about the value to be accorded to his formulae:

> It is clear that it is not because I used a formulation made up of the irruption of mathematics into logic that I use it in quite the same way . . . the way I make use of it is such that it is in no way expressible in terms of the logic of propositions.

Having thus arranged his formulae

$$\begin{array}{ll} \exists x.\overline{\Phi x} & \overline{\exists x}.\overline{\Phi x} \\ \forall x.\Phi x & \overline{\forall x}.\Phi x \end{array},$$

he continues:

> [I]n the two cases, at these two levels (the 'lower' and the 'upper') which are as such independent, and it is not at all a matter of making one the negation of the other, but on the contrary of one an obstacle to the other. . . . Far from one opposing the other as its negation, it is quite the contrary from their subsistence, here very precisely as negated, that there is an x that can be sustained in this beyond of the phallic function. And on the other side, there is not one for the simple reason that a woman cannot be castrated. . . . Far then from the relation of negation forcing us to choose, it is on the contrary that far from having to choose we have to divide up, that the two sides are legitimately opposed one another.

The article by Brunschwig: maximal and minimal particular

So now we have been warned about how futile it would be to make these formulae function as opposing couples, which would *ipso facto* bring back again the original duality from which we are trying to escape. Lacan does not use any microscope to approach masculine and feminine enjoyment in order to write their differential formulae; on the contrary, he attempts to put in peril the (negative) universal which he has been drumming in for a long time as not being suitable to capture in its nets the phallic function as he has fabricated it. We would only have then a partial view of the global operation that he is attempting at the level of this universal, if we were not to enquire in the text that played here, in an undeniable way, the role of source, namely the article by Jacques Brunschwig published in 1969 in No. 10 of the *Cahiers pour l'analyse*, an article titled 'The Particular Proposition and the Proofs of Non-conclusiveness in Aristotle'.[36] Lacan gives the reference, but in going through the sessions where he treats this theme, we see that his debt to Brunschwig is obvious (his references to certain writings of Aristotle in Greek all come from the article).

Brunschwig right away draws attention to the problem linked to the particular proposition in Aristotle: in the natural tongue, it could, in effect, be understood in two different senses, one described as 'maximal' and the other 'minimal', a double meaning that Aristotle notes in his quest aimed at differentiating the forms of syllogism, which allow a conclusion to be drawn in every case, and those that prohibit, just as formally, any valid conclusion whatsoever. How separate them out from one another? Aristotle works on many occasions, either by the 'proof by contrasting instances' or by the 'proof by the indeterminate'.

The two meanings, 'maximal' and 'minimal', are woven into a different rapport of the particular to the universal. When in effect I affirm that 'some A belong to B', two possibilities remain open: either all the A belong to B, in which case it is also true, *a fortiori*, about some, or 'not-all the A belong to B', and in this case, only some belong to it; the others do not belong to it, setting aside with this the truth of the universal affirmative. The first meaning of the particular, which is in agreement with the universal of the same order (affirmative or negative), is said by Brunschwig to be 'minimal' as far as it is but an instantiation of the 'all' of the universal; the second is said to be maximal because it encounters such a maximum below the 'all'. If, in the minimal meaning of the particular, I affirm that 'some A belong to B', then all do; if, on the contrary, I affirm the particular in its maximal meaning, 'some A belong to B', I rule out by this step that 'all' belong to it, only 'not-all' do so (this was the case of the roots of second-degree equations mentioned by Lacan on 19 May 1971).

In following Brunschwig, we see Aristotle getting entangled in the difficulties of his research into procedures which would allow there to be isolated with some certainty the forms of conclusive syllogisms, independently of the concepts applied to them and so then in a sense that we would call today strictly formal. The whole article comes back to showing how, in the course of his work, Aristotle never stopped excluding the maximal sense of the particular, understanding that this meaning generated by itself most of the difficulties that he encountered in his efforts on this point. Brunschwig concludes his demonstrative movement on this point by these lines:

> This clarification of the situation corresponds to a now total liquidation of the maximal connotations of the particular. The 'logical' particular [the 'minimal', the one then at which Aristotle ended up] had some trouble in killing off the 'natural' particular [that of the natural tongue, the 'maximal' which leaves open the two meanings of the particular]; but it ended up by getting there.

How does Brunschwig come to such a conclusion? He cannot content himself with the ambiguity present in language about the 'some' and is compelled to build the logical squares regarding, respectively, minimal and maximal meaning. It is worthwhile following him in his endeavour because of the putting in order of the different propositions, that is the logical square invented long after Aristotle by Apuleius. This square arranges the four places that we have already encountered (*a*, *e*, *i*, *o*), in order, putting on left the affirmative ones, on right the negative ones. The universal ones on the top, the particular ones on the bottom.

The start is now given by this general schema:

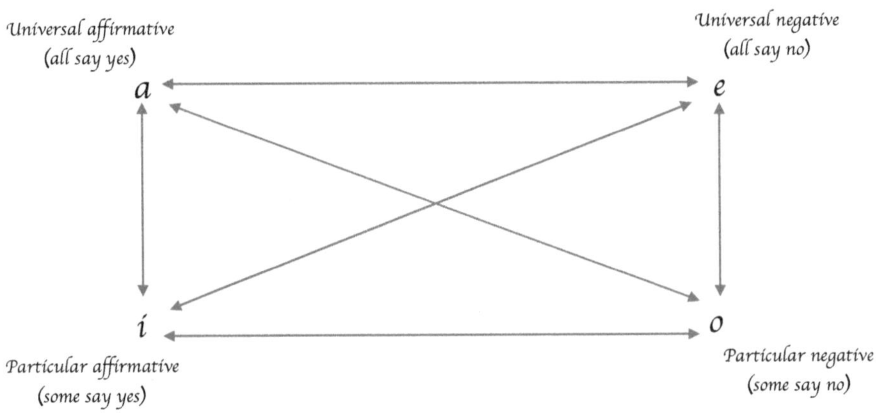

Thanks to this little device of presentation, it is now easier to appreciate the logical consequences of this distinction between the two meanings of the word *some* and the logical squares it generates. If we decide to make clear that the relations between the four terms such as the universal affirmative and the particular affirmative are true at the same time – the 'minimal' case into which *some* is but an instantiation of *all* and has not any restrictive meaning – then it follows that 'some say yes' (that is '*i*') is in contradiction with *e* ('all say no') and is implicated by *a* ('all say yes'), that 'some say no' is in contradiction with '*a*' ('all say yes') and is implicated by *e* ('all say no'), and finally, if 'some say yes', given that 'all say yes', it is excluded that 'some say no'.

The two particular propositions can be true alternatively, or true altogether (but in this case, the two universals are wrong, we will see that better a little further). It is only excluded that they are wrong at the same time; therefore, they are connected by a logical relation named 'compatibility'. We thus get a relation of contradiction between every particular and its opposite universal, a relation of implication between every particular and its universal, and a relation of compatibility between the two particulars. It follows from that that the two universals are, either alternatively true, or wrong at the same time (when the two particulars are true), but under no circumstances can they be true at the same time. They are therefore linked by a relation of contrariety, that leads us to this logical square, the one we will name 'minimal', with its internal relations:

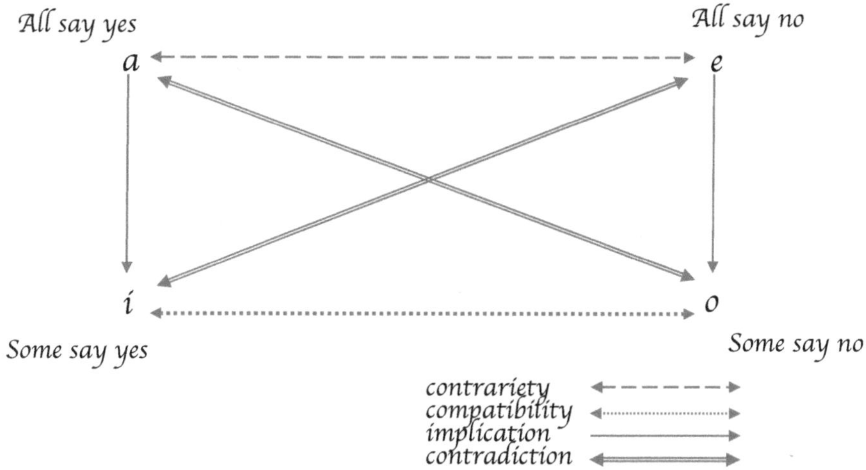

Now, with the other case, the one Brunschwig names 'maximal', into which it is true that 'some say yes', but also, because of the restrictive meaning given straightaway to this meaning, it is excluded by principle that it be the case of 'all', and therefore, it is also necessarily true that 'some say no'. We can see immediately that between the universal affirmative and its particular, there is now necessarily a relation of contradiction; since it is true that, when some say yes, some others say no, it is always wrong that all say yes (it is equally wrong that all say no). The relation of implication that linked universal and particular in the 'minimal' case, now gives room to a relation of contradiction. The previous relation of contradiction between every particular and its opposite universal keeps being valid. We thus come to this new logical square, the one Brunschwig named 'maximal':

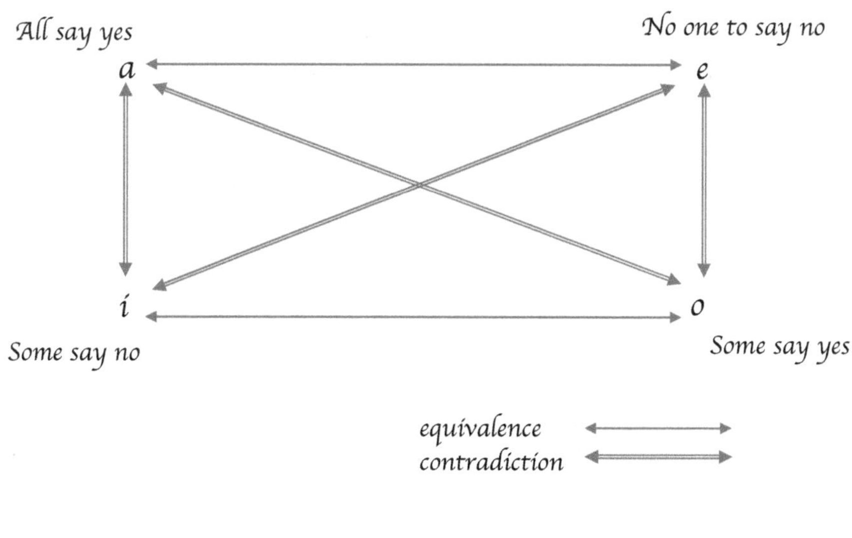

If this 'maximal' square is more in agreement with common language and common sense regarding the particulars, it offends this same common sense with its universals, which, far from being the one the negation of the other, are now in agreement insofar as they say referentially the same thing: 'all say yes', or there is 'no one to say no'; it is all much of a muchness.

The matter becomes clearer a little later, when Brunschwig goes into the details of the proof described as 'by indetermination', in which Aristotle brings the indetermination of the particular, its double maximal/minimal value, into operation in order to manage to settle the doubtful cases of non-conclusiveness, that is when a particular is considered as true and that it is impossible to know if its universal is true or not. Brunschwig writes, to finish with this question:

> One is then logically led to suppose that Aristotle must have sometimes used the indetermination of the particular *without explicitly saying so*; this way of doing things, if it were verified, would allow it to be said this time that the maximal particular is not simply dead, but well and truly buried.[37]

The very technical lines that follow verify this hypothesis, and we then understand that Lacan is striving to take up the challenge of what Aristotle, according to Brunschwig, had to drop in order to make his proofs of non-conclusiveness consistent. Over against the Stagyrite, he finds, in effect, in this 'maximal particular', the instrument which, instead of giving access to a universal 'whole' which embarrasses him in more ways than one, opens up for him the path of a plurality without closure and thus of an existence without essence – the very one that he wants to set off to advantage on the woman side.[38] He very well knows that, in doing so, he is in opposition with the mainstream of logical tradition that follows blindly Aristotle on this point. A very good and recent textbook of standard logic[39] gives a mention of this maximal meaning of the particular only in a little footnote:

> One will pay attention to the fact that natural discourse generally *presupposes* that if 'some F is G', it is excluded that 'all F are G'. That is not the case of Logic that interprets the quantifier $\exists$ as signifying only 'at least one' (F is G), and does not exclude in any sense that 'all' (F are G).

Exit the maximal meaning of the particular, it will no longer be present in the logical calculus.

Lacan and his maximal particular: the 'not-all'

Lacan thus privileges this maximal form of particular which objects to the universal while affirming at the same time that if some x possess the property, one would be wrong to conclude from this that, consequently, they all do. Quite the contrary:

not-all possess it. It is with respect to this that we must again make an effort of comprehension: classically, if not-all possess it and, at the same time, some others do not possess it, the conjunction then of the elements that possess it and of those that do not possess it brings back the whole of the universal. It is here that Lacan intervenes anew to consolidate his not-all with its critical value with respect to the universal. He writes that at the same time, in the right-hand formulae, if not-all possess it, there are none that do not possess it:

$$\overline{\forall x}.\Phi x, \text{then}\, \overline{\exists x}.\overline{\Phi x}$$

Here the not-all reigns in the sense that there is in this respect no x that does not satisfy the function Φ and that nevertheless those which do satisfy it do not constitute the *totality* of elements that satisfy it. Here is the difficulty:[40] to think that there is no exception ($\overline{\exists x}.\overline{\Phi x}$), that there are none to say no, and that nevertheless the collection of those which satisfy, which say yes ($\overline{\forall x}.\Phi x$), does not reunite under the aegis of some universal from which one could draw, in an 'indeterminate' way, an element that one could then inscribe in the particular of the same order. To exemplify by a verb, if not-all say yes, there are none to say no, and of course, there is no question of saying anything other than yes or no;[41] silence here is not an option.

This apparent eccentricity is yet in perfect agreement with the order developed by the maximal proposition such as Lacan takes it from Aristotle, who had abandoned it. When he writes that the two universals, affirmative and negative, far from being contradictory, are equivalent – what C. S. Peirce suggests to him for a long time and that he commented on years ago through the formulae 'all men are liars' ($\forall x.\Phi x$), and 'there is no man no to be a liar' ($\overline{\exists x}.\overline{\Phi x}$) – Lacan follows punctiliously the maximal logical square. This equivalency between the universals, very strange for logic and common sense that largely prefer that universals affirmative and negative be in contradiction, is never the less perfectly regular in the frame of the maximal proposition. There is here nothing coming from the mysteries of femininity.

Lacan ends up then at this apparent paradox that his universal negative is henceforth written with the help of the negation of the existential quantifier ($\overline{\exists x}$), while his particular negative, strictly 'maximal', is written for its part with the help of the negation of the universal quantifier ($\overline{\forall x}$). A way of signifying that the 'not-all' does not allow any 'some' that would contradict it to overlap. The absence of exception that the universal negative affirms in a movement of double negation – at once on the existential quantifier and on the function – is offered as the indispensable complement of a maximal particular, since it contradicts the opposite universal: if 'not-all' say yes ($\overline{\forall x}.\Phi x$), it is ruled out that all should do so or that there should be one who does not do so – because the universal negative affirms it on its side: not one who does not ($\overline{\exists x}.\overline{\Phi x}$).

How can we avoid falling back into the binary?

The core of the operation, both on the left-hand side and the right-hand side (to stop conferring values that are too imaginary by already naming them 'man' and 'woman') is nothing other than the conception of the exception. It is obvious on one side ($\exists x.\overline{\Phi x}$); it is denied on the other ($\overline{\exists x}.\overline{\Phi x}$). Jean-Claude Milner, in his brief commentary on the matter,[42] makes great play of this opposition, without paying too much attention to the fact that just by itself, it reduces the reading of these formulae to a strict binarity, namely, what Lacan is trying to take his distance from.

It is certainly sensible to distinguish as he does the infinite, potentially present in the 'whole', and the unlimited, which possesses a quite different make-up: the surface of a sphere is a finite 'whole' and nevertheless unlimited (without any point or series of points that create a limit); the fragment of a real straight line [0, 1] is a limited whole (a bounded one) and is nevertheless infinite. If Milner had not tried to highlight only this opposite couple for the needs of his argument, the most obscure manual of topology would have furnished him with apt examples. Why then go looking for the Lacan of the formulae of sexuation, if it is only to return to a couple of opposites founded on the presence/absence of a pertinent feature: limited *versus* unlimited? The linguist will perhaps find himself at ease here, but the serious reader of the formulae much less so since he will find himself stuck on a binarity which it was a question of getting rid of.

Good-bye, in that case, to discordance and foreclosure and to the perfectly logical correction of the square produced by Lacan on the basis of Brunschwig's maximal particular! With all the clarity of his relevant feature, Milner rushes towards a suggestion of the same Lacan that we will study much more closely in what follows, namely that the exception might function as 'limit'. This conceptual reduction (exception = limit) suggested by Lacan, just like the example, added on by Milner, of scholastic logic distinguishing between divisible terms and transcendent terms (which do not divide) allows him to give as the ultimate reason for this attack on the univocal nature of the universal . . . a bi-partition which brings back again the universal in all its unbroken splendour. The attack on the universal, to believe him, was only then a strategic ruse, designed to spare a step for local demonstrative ends (to distinguish two alls with different make-ups), without putting in question the sway of the universal.

On the contrary, we have seen that Lacan insists on the fact that it is not a matter of opposing but of 'creating an obstacle' by one to the other, to make them 'subsist' by one another,[43] just as in an Aristotelian logical square the four propositions *a*, *e*, *i*, *o* are sustained together, in an interplay of mutual relations, certainly regulated by dual oppositions and nevertheless irreducible to these latter. It would be well then to approach differently the global consistency of the set of these four formulae if one wants to avoid the trap of reading them as formulae that are fundamentally dualist, right away ready to take on board, under the henceforth impressive colours of logic, the most retrograde opinions about . . . what made them man and woman.

Inversely, before looking for the pertinent feature that would differentiate 'man' and 'woman', Lacan picks out, in Brunschwig's article, what the latter signals as having been rejected by Aristotle, in other words, the maximal particular. He signals this, in his own way and much later, during the first session of the seminar . . . *or Worse*: 'the not-all which is precisely and very curiously what Aristotelian logic eluded'.[44] Nevertheless, to sustain such a rapprochement, it is not enough to be satisfied with just the support taken from the appellation 'not-all' that Brunschwig finds in Aristotle and that Lacan wants to blow up. To convince oneself that what is at stake here is a conceptual and not simply a nominal borrowing, it is necessary to study the logical squares of these two elements: the maximal particular in Aristotle and the final writing of the formulae of sexuation in Lacan. I am helped by the fact that Brunschwig, also careful to give a logical consistency to his remarks, offers to differentiate the minimal and the maximal for us by their profoundly different logical squares (he even offers himself the luxury of constructing a third, 'for recreational purposes').

The logical square of the maximal particular

It is sufficient to set the writings proposed by Lacan to realise that they fit exactly with the logical square of the maximal: the universal affirmative $\forall x.\Phi x$ and the universal negative $\overline{\exists x}.\overline{\Phi x}$ are in contradiction with their opposite particulars, respectively, $\exists x.\overline{\Phi x}$ and $\overline{\forall x}.\Phi x$, while universals are linked by equivalence, as particulars also do. In these conditions, what about the logical square proposed by Lacan, even he does not take the trouble to construct it as such? It can be depicted as follows:

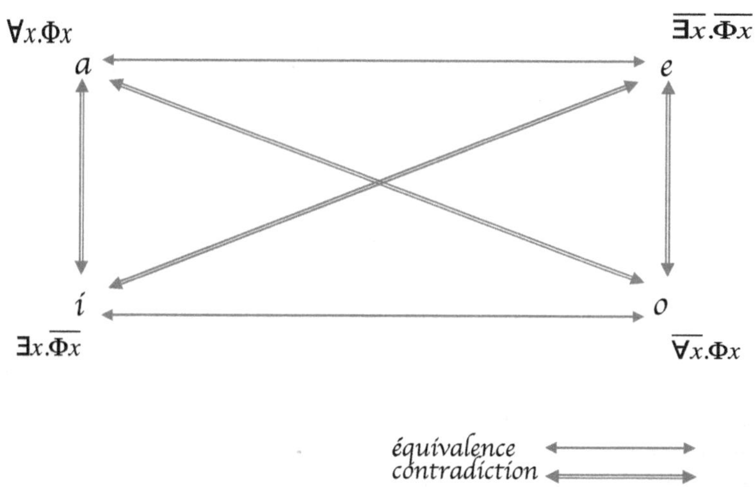

As this writing makes visible, *a* enters into contradiction both with *i* and with *o* (if all say yes, then it is false both that one says no and that not all say yes); in the same way *e* enters into contradiction with *i* and *o* (if there are none to say no, then it is false both that there is one who says no and that not all say yes) Moreover, the two universals imply one another since, if all say yes, this in no way enters into contradiction, or even contrariety, with the fact that none says no. In the same way, the two particulars are implied by one another: that there should be some who say no remains congruent with the fact that not all say yes.

This construction for the moment has only one interest: to bring out that this logical square is the one that Brunschwig constructs to explicate the maximal particular. In effect, he writes in this connection:

> The two particulars are implied by one another; if one wants the couples *a-o* and *e-i* to remain contradictory, one is paradoxically led to admit that each of the particulars, on the one hand exclude the universal of the same quality, and is excluded by it, on the other hand continues to exclude the universal of the opposite quality and to be excluded by it; in effect, each of the universals cannot contradict one particular without contradicting the other, which is equivalent to it. It follows moreover that the two universals are now equivalent, because they contradict two equivalent propositions.[45]

What is at stake then is indeed the same arrangement as in the logical square of the formulae of sexuation. With this concordance, we have the proof that the rapprochement between what was scrapped by Aristotle and discovered by Lacan is valid. And nevertheless, what Lacan was trying to make of it is not so easily deduced; this cocking a snoot at Aristotle, this explicit wish to bring out the 'problem' linked to the universal, certainly originates in this decision to take up the challenge of the maximal particular but just as much in the fact of being willing to fight for something well beyond this fencing of logicians.

Why cannot Lacan be satisfied by the simple maximal particular so well isolated by Brunschwig? If such had been the case, it would have been enough to refer to it! Now the reasons he has to go looking on this side of things – namely to make the meaning of the universal negative vacillate to stop having to deal with 'all men' versus 'all women' – push him a little further. It is clear, in effect, that, if the maximal particular poses for Aristotle problems of logical consistency in his proofs of non-conclusiveness, it does not lead just by itself to a new status of the universal negative – which Lacan always wants to put in place. How?

To understand it, we must now become attentive to the *movement of the writing* of the four formulae that compose his logical square. Lacan starts, like everybody else, from the universal affirmative which he writes then: $\forall x.\Phi x$. His choice of the maximal particular, and his concern to produce the three other formulae with the operator of a redoubled negation (the 'strong' and the 'weak', like Blanché), leads him at first to affirm the particular negative by sustaining the existence of 'not-all', in other words, already, to write a particular by putting a negation on the universal operator ($\overline{\forall x}.\Phi x$). Writing the particular affirmative, Lacan should then in this respect (as Blanché suggests) write $\overline{\forall x}.\overline{\Phi x}$. For reasons that will appear later (with the word *exception*), Lacan transforms what is called the weak negation of the universal quantifier ($\overline{\forall x}$), into an existential quantifier ($\exists x$), thus producing for the writing of the particular affirmative $\exists x.\overline{\Phi x}$. In this substitution, *not all* is held to be equivalent to *some*, and with that, the particular affirmative unveils something of the regular handling of writing by Lacan: it first writes the *maximal* meaning by affirming, not that there are some to illustrate the affirmative universal (which would remain ambiguous) but that there are some who do *not* illustrate it, because of *not* going in its direction. This decision – inconceivable in Brunschwig/Aristotle, for whom the maximal particular and the 'some, but not all' is *read* in the relations of the logical square but is *not written at its* place – is going to shift everything.

There remains in effect the thorny problem of the writing of the universal negative. According to Blanché, it should be written *universally not-p*, in other words: $\forall x.\overline{\Phi x}$. Now this does not at all suit Lacan, who is trying to evacuate the whole dimension of universality in his formulae on the right (that began right away with the 'not-all'[46] of the particular negative). He applies then the inverse solution to the one that has just allowed him to write a particular (negative) with the negation of the universal quantifier; he is now going to write a universal quantifier by denying an existential quantifier. Instead of $\forall x$, he writes: $\overline{\exists x}$. Are these inversions between quantifiers legitimate? Can we go from the one to the other by simple negation?

Logically, there is room to doubt it. That the negation of universality should produce existence is already questionable: if 'not all', then 'some', certainly, but I can just as well sustain 'if not all, then none'. And in the same way, if I affirm: 'not some', I can just as well conclude 'then all' as 'then none'. An essential ambiguity is here renewed in this writing operation, which has nothing anodyne about it.

Now this ambiguity is what Lacan has been aiming at for more than ten years already, since the session of the seminar *Identification* in the course of which he saluted Peirce's intuition according to which the universal negative can be conceived not simply as the set of elements which do not satisfy the function but also as the locus where no element is met with. The 'not some' ($\overline{\exists x}$) *is* to be read as 'none', even while it is taking the place of an 'all'. This indeed is the step that Lacan takes with his writing of the universal negative: $\overline{\exists x}.\overline{\Phi x}$: there are none to say no.

Here, undeniably, is situated the high point of his invention, much more than on the side of the 'not-all' (Aristotle, relayed by Brunschwig, had already proposed it) or of the apparent contradiction between the universal and particular affirmative (which only stems from the maximal meaning of the particular proposition). For in deciding to write the universal negative by the negation of an existential quantifier, Lacan rejoins the intuition of Peirce to better anchor his subject, which, we have seen him argue, maintain a very special rapport with the nothing, a nothing different to that of Freud or Hegel.[47] But above all, with this writing he secures a sort of bolting down of his battery of formulae which, otherwise, would go down the tubes.

In effect, the 'not-all' of the particular negative should not be read as 'some', as a partitive which would allow us to think that, if some say yes (just as on the left, some say no), the others say no (as on the left, the others, those of the all which are not the some, say yes). Here, Lacan only wants to break the symmetry, and he does it with his writing of the universal negative which affirms that none say no, there where, precisely, 'not all' say yes. The fact is that here, on the right, the 'not all' should not be understood as a partitive but as the affirmation that the elements present on this side are each subject to the same regime, without nevertheless ever being the elements of any 'all'.[48] Their existence under this regime of the phallic function does not lead them to make a set, leaves them loose, in an existence unattached to any essence within which these elements would be subsumed: that is what had to be put down in black-and-white, to be produced in its logical consistency, ever since the critical reading of the myth of 'all the women' in *Totem and Taboo*.

The logical square developed by Lacan is then indeed that of the maximal particular, but it is written in such a way, with this inversion of universal and existential quantifiers, that it presents in the writing of each proposition the logical fault (*faille*) that the particular in the Brunschwig style did not allow to be read except in the unfolding of relations internal to the logical square. By reason of these formulae, he ensures that the left side and the right side do not present a mirror consistency, can no longer be opposed in a perfect symmetry but contribute reciprocally to one another obstacle and support. By doing this, Lacan shows that he is aware of the fact that if one wants to undermine the dualities Man/Woman, Yin/Yang, XX/XY, penised/un-penised, and so on, one must not hesitate to damage their logical underpinnings, since he is sure that logic, in its own foundation, is much more 'gendered' (because of its fundamental binarity) than 'sexed'. It is important to be convinced of this point, otherwise one will miss the intuition that pushes him to bring together 'logical fault' and 'sexual fault'. For him, sex touches on logic, but logic touches just as much on sex. So that reconnecting them with one another illuminates the one and the other, the one by the other, while the couples of opposites sustain logics of the kind (man/woman, active/passive, etc.) which, for their part, seek to articulate themselves without fault, and without remainder.

It is no longer very difficult, starting from this reading, to locate the connecting point by which Lacan assumes the authority to join together logic and sex in a sort of fault that if not common, is at least close. The attentive reader of the seminar *From an Other to the Other* can know that what Lacan retains in Russell's paradox, is the inexistence of a set which, at first sight, appears to be just as well made as any other: the set of all the sets that do not belong to themselves. Through this fault that he found in Frege's *Foundations of Arithmetic*, Russell had opened up the crisis about foundations in mathematics. What Lacan is attempting on the right side of the formulae is of the same order. He no more denies the existence of each woman than Russell (or anyone else) would have the notion of denying that there exist sets that do not belong to themselves. The problem is that no set collectivises them. It is not a matter then, at the point to which Lacan is trying to bring his listeners of that time, of finding THE pertinent feature that would allow Man and Woman to be correctly ranked in their respective sets – since then it would be really child's play to write their 'rapport' – but to make appear between them an irreducible asymmetry which does not depend on any feature given from elsewhere.[49] This alone will offer its chance to the non-rapport.

Milner's approach in his latest work is therefore not destined to have a great future for anyone who is trying to read these formulae of sexuation, for the good and simple reason that he only reads there what is important to him: to distinguish two 'alls'. If what differentiates on the side of man and on the side of women these formulae of sexuation proved to be only the presence/absence of a relevant feature (limited versus unlimited), then our customary bipartitions would continue to distribute their places in function of our prejudices about having/not having, castrated/not castrated, active/passive, and so on.[50] The most 'natural' psychology would come then to range itself under the sophisticated banner of these logical formulae, in order to predicate anew essences that their very differences would put '*en rapport*' with one another.

Essence *versus* existence

In cursorily reading the seminars that hash and rehash the formulae of sexuation, we see Lacan returning on several occasions to a distinction that he is fond of: being (essence) *versus* existence. The inexistence of the sexual rapport stems, first of all, from the fact of deconstructing essences, of recognising that it is not possible to produce symbols at the same level on the side of man and on the side of woman (except by considering both one and the other as essences each developed by a consistent universal, which he precisely wants to deny). Because for him, as for everyone, the 'for any', the ∀ of modern logic is directed at being and essence: once I say, and especially when I write 'any man', I produce one of these 'semi-twilight entities' (as W. V. O. Quine called them), a pure symbol whose denotation is waiting to be effectuated and which by this fact does not establish any existence but produces a being that can be qualified and thus an essence. Inversely, the 'there exists' (∃) shows its hand since it says what it is doing: it right away asserts the existence of the element that it writes. The problem for Lacan, is that without taking extra precautions, this existence right away accompanies an essence, always finds itself in relation with the supposition of the being of the universal, which is illustrated by the minimal particular to which Aristotle retreats since, with it, existence is never anything but the singular actualisation of a being always universal in its category. Here is what Lacan, for multiple reasons that, in part, go beyond the business of the sexual rapport, rejects, to the extent of sometimes speaking about what Aristotle 'missed' by operating in this way (that Brunschwig has suggested to him). Now, an existence without essence, or which at least is posited outside any necessity of an essence of its own, is what Lacan has been on the trail of since he put the partial of the 0-object into orbit, and which has continued in the epic of 'There is no sexual *rapport*'. His insistence on existence does not rank him that much amongst structuralists than on the side of existentialists, not in the style of Sartre or Mousnier but in the line of descent which, from Pascal to Kierkegaard passing by Maine de Biran, want in different ways to make existence prevail over essence, in a tenacious struggle against the dominant philosophical tradition which is, always, that of the concept first.

3 March 1972: the exception proves the rule

On this point, we must now closely follow the sharp turn that he initiates on 3 March 1972, a session to be marked in red for what we are concerned with here in the measure that it is, by far, one of the richest on the subject. He is conscious of this:

> Here I am bringing forward a glimpse that is lacking to the function, to the notion of species and of class. It is in this sense that it is not by chance that this whole dialectic was missed out in the Aristotelian forms.

Since what is at stake is to make the universal vacillate, to disconnect it from its adherence to an all into which one would only have to dip to obtain any element whatsoever, Lacan is going to have to work twice as hard in the measure that he is going to have to produce, in each deixis,[51] an element capable of contravening Aristotle's way of tying things up by trying to derive existence from essence. This 3 March seminar, he begins with the man side:

> Where finally does there function this $\exists x.\overline{\Phi x}$, this 'there-exists-at-least-one' who is not the slave of the phallic function? It is only from a requisite, I would say of a type that is despairing from the point of view of something that is not even supported by a universal definition. But on the contrary note that with regard to the Universal marked by $\forall x.\Phi x$ every male is a slave of the phallic function. What is meant then by the 'at least one' as functioning to escape from it? I would say that it is the exception. It is indeed the occasion when what is said, without knowing what it says, the proverb that 'the exception confirms the rule'[52], is there to support us. It is curious that it is only with the analytic discourse that a Universal can find, in the existence of the exception, its true foundation which ensures that undoubtedly we can in any case distinguish the Universal thus grounded from any use rendered commonplace by the philosophical tradition of the aforesaid Universal.

Here then we have henceforth acknowledged Lacan's ambition in logic: to *found a new universal on the exception that objects to it.* We begin to guess here the benefit he has gained by first of all splitting the bar of negation and by ensuring that the two particulars, the 'positive' and the 'negative', both enter into contradiction with each universal (in this case equivalent, as we have just seen). This clearly signifies that if the particulars are true (Lacan is going to make sure that the balance tips to this side), the two universals are necessarily false, and one must be able to tolerate working within a permanent contradiction between the level of universals where essences and concepts are formulated, and the level of particulars where existences are affirmed as such.

In the measure nevertheless that the famous proverb which would make of the exception the confirmation of the universal does not throw any light likely to instruct us in the matter, we must indeed accept, at the point that we are at in it, that this support for the universal by the exception remains mysterious – this is the reason why we will soon enquire about the state of exception to glean some light with respect to this, because what Lacan is able at this time to articulate about the opposition man/woman is not going to illuminate us on the relevance of his formal effort to damage the universal as all.

The important thing for the moment, in the obscurity in which we find ourselves as regards the meaning to give to this unusual value (in logic) of the exception, is to see in detail how Lacan argues his point in the other deixis, on the right-hand side. In effect, he takes care – it is one of the two formulae – to write in black-and-white that here there is no exception: $\overline{\exists x}.\overline{\Phi x}$.

> This is something that has no parallel, symmetry with the requirement that I called earlier 'despairing' of the 'at least one'. . . . The fact that there is no exception does not any more assure the Universal that is already so badly established by reason of the fact that it is discordant, does not assure anymore the Universal of the woman. The 'without exception', far from giving to some 'All' a consistency, naturally gives still less to what is defined as 'not all'.[53]

This 'naturally' is just as valid as the '*naturlich*' that we find here and there in Freud: it signals a real perplexity, and in fact, in reading these seminars, the dominant impression with respect to the junction of the 'not-all' to the woman results more from a repetition than from a clarification. What emerges on the contrary from this half-darkness, is the fact that where no exception is conceived of, the all is nonetheless denied by the quantifier 'not-all'.

The only possible way of comprehending this sort of passionate and tautological affirmation of Lacan in this respect is once again mathematical and logical: there is a decisive difference between a set of individuals and the domain that they constitute. In the first, they make a 'set'. They are taken up into a unity of which they are the elements. In this respect, either they *belong* or they are *included* in the aforesaid set. The domain would be something like the same elements, but not collectivised, which would neither belong to nor be included in any 'set' whatsoever.[54] This is what Lacan aspires to write with a domain of individuals whose existence one affirms at the same time (thanks to the negation of the universal quantifier, $\overline{\forall x}$, valid here as an existential quantifier) but that one refuses to collectivise since the exclusion of the exception amounts to affirming that there is not, on this side, any who escape the 'not-all', *without this absence of exception bringing about a closure for all that.* With these two contradictory formulae, conjoined in the same deixis, Lacan posits a domain of individuals escaping any collectivisation that would produce an essence of them, as well as the definite article which, in French, is the sign of it, hence the famous 'The woman does not exist', a provocative residual statement from this search for the missing universal in the speaking being and this 'The' pointing to a naturally supposed 'set' of women than would give room to an essence of 'woman', which is here denied again.

Let us summarise so as to be able to render simultaneously present to our minds the irreducibly plural elements of the kind of bifid point on which Lacan's logical square rests: *on left side, inasmuch as there is an all, it is founded on the existence of the exception of at least one (therefore possibly some or several), and on right side, inasmuch as there is no exception, the several (some, 'not-all') that exist do not form any all.* In both cases, the universal no longer holds up as collecting, without exception, all the elements which, through belonging or through inclusion, would give rise to a compact and homogenous unity. It is always the same attack by Lacan against the encompassing all which he had, from his first seminars, hooked onto the specular image, and which he rediscovers here under the form of the universal. The partiality of the object, as quite clearly since the seminars *Transference* and *Identification*, claims its due here by requiring that something exists that cannot be brought back to belonging to or inclusion in a universal.

We will not ask here whether this logical equilibrium is congruent or not with the difference of the sexes or the impossibility of the sexual rapport. We will be content to remark that the universal (that there is no question of doing without; it is what allows us to write with complete security) maintains with the exception a relationship that Lacan to my mind, does not manage to clarify in the course of these two seminars, *Of a Discourse That Might Not Be a Semblance* and *. . . or Worse.* To stick to the formulae in their final state, far from rushing to split them into two sides (whatever name one bestowed on them) to better charge each one with 'its' own contradiction, it is better to try to hold them together; it is only from this angle that we manage to make ourselves sensitive to the repetition of the contradiction without which Lacan's whole effort is there and then brought back to ancestral and ideologically weighty truths concerning the difference between the genders (let us no longer even talk about sex in this climb-down to the bipolar). On the left, in effect, the particular objects to its universal, just the same as on the right, but each side also objects to the other in that one affirms the existence of the exception, while the other denies it. So then we have to settle the fragile status of this contradiction with regard to the exception, in one way or another, since it is offered as the keystone of this little pyramid which consists only in producing two types of contradiction (one proper to each deixis and the other between the deixis).

On the exception conceived of as a limit

The only effective help that Lacan brings us in this maze is to be found, not in the seminars, but in the text published in Scilicet, then in *Autres écrits*, in which he argues:

> The second [we are dealing with the 'second writing' with respect to the $\forall x.\Phi x$], [in other words the $\exists x.\overline{\Phi x}$], there is exceptionally the case, familiar in mathematics, (the argument $x = 0$ in the hyperbolic function $1/x$), the case where there exists an x for which Φx, the function is not satisfied, namely, since it does not function, is de facto excluded.[55]

A hyperbolic function of the kind $1/x$ is presented as follows:

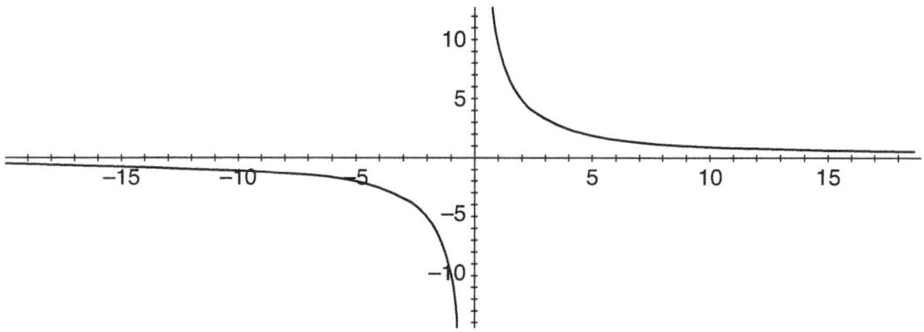

The value 0 is a 'limit'[56] for the curve in the sense that the function tends towards the infinite while the x tends towards zero (and tends towards zero when x tends towards infinity), but no longer presents any value if $x = 0$ since the operation of division can in no way be sustained if one wants to divide any number whatsoever by 0. Lacan therefore situates his $\exists x.\overline{\Phi x}$ at the locus and the place of zero in the hyperbolic function, which underpins very well on the visual plane, his idea that the universal, the for-any (*pourtout*) should take its support on the exception, which, despite the very apparent contradiction, offers it a 'foundation'. The trouble in this example is the profound disparity between the curve and the coordinate axes, the perfect exteriority, in principle, between the coordinate axes and a curve, whatever it may be.

Here again we are brought to a halt on the point of the question posed by Lacan with his formulae: Is the limit to be included in the set, as can be the case in a topological figure which includes its bound, or is it to be excluded from the set, as is suggested (a little too strongly) by the example of the hyperbola in which the value $x = 0$, in other words, the y-axis, does not belong at any point to the curve $y = 1/x$?

In a certain way, we have the answer, even though Lacan does not articulate it in any way, to the best of my knowledge, in the course of the seminars that we have been focusing on. We have the answer because, if the limit should be thought of as exterior to the series (which, then, the $y = 1/x$ suggests), it would risk very quickly becoming transcendent. Since St Anselm (and even St Augustine), there have been no lack of attempts to position God as the superior element, exterior to the worldly series. Where, in effect, must one place oneself to see both the series and its limit, if the latter is to be thought of as exterior to the series, if not in the position of the believer whose faith authorises him to make the most of a . . . revelation? Religion is never very far from this intellectual elegance which wants to arrange with equal certainty both its knowledge and what constitutes its limit.

Another argument: where the exception is excluded, on the right-hand side of the formulae, the all does not manage to be founded, which retroacts on each element by spoiling its unity since it proves to be only an existence without essence.

The right thing to do is then to think of the absence of exception without taking, here either, the point of view from which it would become possible to see the series and then something that does not belong to the series, in order to subsequently pronounce on the fact that this series, decidedly, does not possess a limit while the other, yes, does.

To set off to advantage – as Lacan sustains – existence over essence is to prohibit for oneself any cosmic viewpoint at any given time. To be coherent with what leads him to support the non-rapport, we must then try to think of the exception *starting from the series* (this does not mean that it belongs to it) and not in a space that would include both the series and its exception/limit. The little word *despairing* that Lacan used to indicate from where might come such a *petitio principii*, suitable for positing the existence of an exception, said clearly, in its way, a little psychologically, that it is the 'any *x*' who envisages the exception and not some demiurge fashioning from the mud the humanity that he wants to fabricate or some totemic father choosing at will from his fish pond of women. Except that if we remain with this, the exception is no longer anything but a wish, religious in style, clearly worthy of this hope for an eternal life that we must sometimes be prepared to hear about at funerals: since this exception-in-chief Jesus rose from the dead, all (his faithful) one by one, will have a right to do so. The exception, in this perspective, is no longer anything but the matter of a common future. I strongly doubt that Lacan meant it in this way so that his 'despairing', which refers back to his reading of *Totem and Taboo*, is not something on which one can take support for long to receive the status of exception that he proposes with his formulae of sexuation, which alone sustain with some rigour the sexual non-rapport which for the moment we are concerned with.

To attempt to respond to this difficulty that Lacan situates by his formulae, but leaves in the shadows with just this notion of 'limit', we must part company with him for the moment, and see what happens in other forms of knowledge (*savoirs*) when they find themselves confronted with this same question – which is not proper to the sexes and their difference, but also traverses certain fields of knowledge when they are led to think about what would be radically Other for them. Thus, towards the end of the 19th century, the German scholar du Bois-Reymond wanted to take account of the fact that something always escapes scientific knowledge and had in consequence launched his celebrated '*Ignorabimus*' to which David Hilbert had replied, from the heights of his all-conquering rationalism: 'There is no *ignorabimus*', counting at that time on a demonstration of the non-contradiction of arithmetic which was supposed to guarantee the coherence of scientific thought – nothing less. Godel's theorem, which contradicts him on this crucial point, did not nevertheless in any way justify du Bois-Reymond but demonstrated an entirely new fact: the internal limitation of formalisms because the fields of knowledge that progress by themselves in a rather tentacular fashion only see their consistency specified by the study of their conditions at the limits, as is said about physical systems.[57]

Return to the non-rapport

That the exception exists *and* does not exist, that there is a universal *and* that there is not one, that they can be called 'man' *and* 'woman' insofar as both are ruled by the same function called 'phallic', all of this is only thinkable in the idea, the perspective, the suspicion of non-rapport. Naturally, to think, to speak, to write, is to indefinitely create rapports. And if the order of reasons is shown to be rather parsimonious, indeed fussy for whoever would be more demanding, the signifying rapport, as Lacan had unleashed it by his definition of the subject, is, for its part omnidirectional. There is no internal limitation to specify in advance what signifiers represent the subject for what other signifiers. This restriction would not in truth have any meaning since the definition proposes, among other things, to welcome the 'any' with open arms: any signifier whatsoever is fine for it, it will not quibble. It is far from the idea so dear to the clinician, of generating contraindications and producing a subclass of signifiers which, for their part, would not have the vocation of representing the subject for others. '*Cuentame tu vida*' says a psychoanalytic Argentinean tango, but the definition of the Lacanian subject, which is in perfect agreement with the fundamental Freudian rule, immediately goes well beyond life, biography, and its avatars. Only the unrealisable 'say whatever occurs to you' would be equal to such a definition.

In such a setting, non-rapport is the white blackbird, the 'radical unthought' as it would have been called in an epoch which is growing distant to the point of being today almost past. And the least troubling is not that Lacan had conceived it in his way very early on, from the end of the 1950s, during the elaboration of his 'graph of desire'. In effect, we see appearing there the notation S(s;/) commented on as 'the signifier lacking to the Other'. How can a signifier be lacking to the Other, unequivocally defined at that time, as 'the treasury of signifiers'? Might there not be here something like the beginnings of the exception that we find much later in the form of $\exists x.\overline{\Phi x}$? A question that finds the start of an answer in the very notation of the subject: s;/ which is read as the bar falling on the letter S, up to then appointed to designate the signifier. The subject is not then a signifier but, yes, is indeed what is lacking to the Other, where all the signifiers are collected. The attentive reader of Lacan also knows that this Other, so decisive in the whole theoretical construction 'does not exist', something which cannot be said (by saying it, I *ipso facto* make it exist), but on the other hand can be written: A;/. All these bars brought to bear on letters thus participate in the same movement: One affirms the universal (A: one cannot do better), then one denies it: a;/. Why this passion for erasing?

Because two things must be sustained at once, if not at the same time nor under the same rapport: that the *indefiniteness* of putting into rapport does not raise anything about an abrupt absence of rapport, an absence already highlighted, in a timid and elliptical fashion, by the *leer Gegenstand ohne Begriff*, the empty object without a concept – an object of which I can certainly forge for myself a generic concept (Kant offers it to me ready for use), but under which no worldly object will come to shelter. This 'rose from no bouquet' has the vocation of gullying the signifying circuit, without ever appearing in it as such. We are no longer too surprised, then, to see this contradiction installed at the centre of the writing of the phantasy, in this stamp which at the same time unites (alienation) and disunites (separation) the subject s;/ conceived of as the exception, the $\exists x.\overline{\Phi x}$ able to sustain, like Epimenides that, yes, $\forall x.\Phi x$, and the 0-object as that with which . . . there is no rapport. The sexes come to re-mark this fault, without us knowing too well whether it is because of them, or they because of it.

Addendum

The text you have just read takes up again, from the seminars, the elements that Lacan gathered together in his ultra-cryptic *écrit* published in number 4 of his review Scilicet under the title of *L'Étourdit*. This to say that the reader is invited to read and reread these extremely dense lines with the tone of a last will and testament. But where? Today two publications are offered in the French tongue (we do not dare to invoke the existing translations, given the nature of the source text): the original in *Scilicet*, faulty at least in the quantifiers since, instead of ∀ and ∃, we find, for some mentions of the formulae, A and E, which makes reading it awkward, or the more recent, published in 2000 by Seuil under the general title of *Autres écrits*. Let us choose newness and focus first on this latest publication.

The authority of the printed word having its effect, everything seems to go well . . . until the arrival of the formulae. The bottom of page 458 lets us know in effect about the existence of $\forall x.\Phi x$ and $\exists x.\overline{\Phi x}$. We might regret our refusal to forgive the editor for this V instead of ∀, if the following sentence did not introduce a real difficulty for the novice reader of Lacanisms:

> The first [i.e. the first formula, that written $Vx.\Phi x$, for any x, $Vx.\Phi x$ is satisfied], which can be expressed by a V noting the truth value . . .

Despite this sentence, the V, the classical anagram for the truth value (T in English) is in no way to be confused with the quantifier 'for any', ∀, and it would have been better to follow *Scilicet* which contents itself with writing: $\forall x.\Phi x$. That Lacan is happy here to bring together ∀ and V is not an index of any confusion on his part. A little irritated at this benign error, we are startled when, a few lines further on (on top of page 459), we read the following:

> I combine them because the *There exists one* in question, by creating a limit for the *pourtant* is what affirms or confirms it . . .

It is a matter no doubt of creating a limit for the 'for-any' (*pourtout*) and not for the 'nevertheless' (*pourtant*). What good are the italics that incite the reader to focus his attention a little if the editor himself does not pay any attention to them? A little after the middle of this same page 459, we read:

> It is then correct to write as I do: $\exists x.\Phi x$.

Surprise! Lacan almost never uses this formula but indeed the one that we have encountered on many occasions, that is $\exists x.\overline{\Phi x}$. Does the published text signal a switch as compared to the seminars? The following sentence:

> The one that exists is the subject supposed because the phallic function is missing here (*y fasse forfait*).

The simple word *forfait* removes the hesitation since this writing of the particular affirmative reposes on a type of negation which we have seen Lacan placed on the side of'foreclosure'. He remembers it here with this *forfait*. This forgetting forces the reader then to insert, on his own authority, the bar of negation over Φx. Otherwise, he (the reader) goes off into speculations which, with regard to such a complex text, will rapidly lead him into quicksand. On page 465 is again a surprise. We read:

> That the subject can here propose itself to be called woman depends on two modes. Here they are:
>
> $\overline{\mathrm{E}\, x}.\overline{\Phi x}$ and $\overline{\mathrm{A}\, x}.\Phi x$
>
> Their inscription is not used in mathematics. To deny, as the bar placed above the quantifier marks, to deny that there exists one is not done, and still less that forany gives fornotany (*pourtout se pourpastoute*).

Why then have the letters previously used for quantifiers disappeared to give place to the capitals E and A which already adorned the pages of Scilicet at this place? Has Lacan innovated once again without warning us? Or perhaps he has warned us in his own way in the intervening pages, and it went over our heads? How can we know? But no, in carefully rereading, it seems that nothing of the kind has changed.

Almost all the errors mentioned earlier fall within the competence of a professional proofreader. Why should Jacques Lacan, as an author, not have a right to the usual regime?

But the worst had happened many pages earlier, page 458. When J. C. Milner wants to refer to this passage of *L'Étourdit*, in his work on *The Criminal Leanings of Democratic Europe*, here is how he is obliged to mention his reference: ('an example of Lacan's, *Autres écrits*, p. 458, to be corrected in the light of *Scilicet*, p. 15'). Milner is very kind (even though not to his reader), because the version in *Scilicet* is itself faulty. What does it say?

> [T]here is by exception the case, familiar in mathematics (the argument $x = 0$ in the exponential function $1/\chi$), the case where there exists an x for which Φx, the function, is not satisfied, namely not functioning, is de facto excluded.

Where does this χ come from? Is it Cantor's aleph? But in that case, such writing indexes a number and in no case a function! Can it be said that χ (aleph) is only a rather special writing of 'x'? But then where does there stop the gentle distortion of letters that are supposed to guarantee rigour in calculation? In any case, there is an error, and *Autres écrits*, conscious of the problem, sets out to remedy it. So then it offers the reader the following:

> [T]he argument $x = 0$ in the exponential function x/χ . . .

We immediately feel that if there is progress, it is in the dimension of error, for it is certain that the value $x = 0$ satisfies the function and does not act as a limit to anything, since 0 in the numerator is always acceptable, whatever is in the denominator (except 0).

This little procession of errors – those of *Scilicet*, those of *Autres écrits* which adds a very elementary mathematical ineptitude – allows there to be glimpsed still another error, imputable for its part to none other than Jacques Lacan: why does he here name 'exponential' what is, in fact, a 'hyperbolic' function? An exponential function, which is written e^x, will take on for the value $x = 0$ (like every number that is raised to the power of 0) the value of 1, without encountering here any limit or exception. By taking a slightly critical look, we would have realised what Lacan was alluding to here, and have found (as Milner does on his own account), the writing $1/x$ which, in effect, allows there to be brought together exception and limit for $x = 0$.

Notes

1 In everything that follows, a capital in 'Man' or 'Woman' will designate the concept in its essence, over against 'man' or 'woman' which refer to individuals.
2 J. Lacan, *Desire and Its Interpretation*, unpublished seminar, 29 April 1959. Translated by Cormac Gallagher.
3 J. Lacan, *Object Relations and Freudian Structures*, untranslated seminar, 28 November 1956.
4 Namely, *The Family* (1938), unpublished translation by Cormac Gallagher.
5 In fact, in 1971 in the course of the seminar . . . *or Worse.*
6 I have tried to diversify and to explicate this vocabulary in *Le Lasso spéculaire, une étude traversière de I'unité imaginaire*, Paris, EPEL, 1997.
7 In this, close to the phoneme attached to the linguistic concept of 'pertinence', which makes of it an indivisible unity.
8 J. Lacan, *Transference*, unpublished translation by Cormac Gallagher, 1 February 1961.
9 K. Abraham, *Selected Papers on Psychoanalysis*, London, Maresfield Reprints, 1979, p. 490. Lacan gives a quite special place to the case from which Abraham constructed this notion of 'partial love of the object' during the final sessions of the seminar on *Transference*, while he is elaborating its 'specular dynamics'. The case is that of a female patient dreaming about her naked father without pubic hair (so then an incomplete specular image).

10 That the total object was only one object among others does not seem to have been exploited by Melanie Klein. This nevertheless appears to be a very remarkable intuition.
11 Lacan, *Transference*, 1 February 1961.
12 Something like the obscure link proposed by Peirce in his triadic concept of the sign, between the immediate object (which belongs to the sign) and the dynamic object (which belongs to the world).
13 *Cf. infra*, note 18.
14 I. Kant, *Critique of Pure Reason*, translated by N. K. Smith, London, Macmillan, 1933, pp. 295–296.
15 The words between [] are mine. GLG.
16 Kant, *Critique of Pure Reason, op. cit.*, p. 295.
17 Lacan had previously defined, in a table of his own, three types of object: that of *frustration*, that of *privation* (certainly at the origin of this *ens privativum*), and that of *castration* which is that aimed at by this new look 'partial'.
18 We can also divine from this that the 'we analysts' that curiously punctuates many of the quotations that we have just read, designates rather . . . the other analysts, those whom Lacan intends to oppose with his invention, those who have understood nothing about Freud's inspired 'partial', who are mistaken about the nothing, and so forth.
19 It is a matter of founding a new 'ir-rational', since the word signifies precisely 'non-rapport'. Except that since the advances of Dedekind in *Numbers: What Are They and What Use Are They?* the irrationals are integrated, as organised 'cuts' in the body of real numbers and therefore maintain rapports of order with all the other numbers. They are no longer 'irrational' except in name, and with whole numbers and the rationals (as well as the transcendentals), they form the 'numerical continuum', which has henceforth taken over from the geometrical continuum. Lacan can no longer, then, base himself in any way on and the diagonal of the $\sqrt{2}$ square to get across the 'without-rapport' of his partial. Bye-bye, Meno!
20 J. Lacan, *On a Discourse That Might Not Be a Semblance*, 17 February 1971, unpublished translation by Cormac Gallagher.
21 *Ibid.*, p. 15.
22 Twice, first in *Totem and Taboo* and again in *Moses and Monotheism*, Freud uses the adjective *all* for the women in so far as they are supposed to be the possession of the chief of the horde. But this feature in no way constitutes for him the axis of the affair and is both times taken up in the reference to Darwin who, for his part, affirms that the chief of the horde had appropriated all the women (*sich alle Weibchen aneignete*) S. Freud, *Der Man Moses und die Monotheistiche Religion*, Studienausgabe, vol. 9, Frankfurt, Fischer, 1974, p. 575. In *Totem and Taboo*, the unique mention of this point is found in Darwin's quotation (in English SE XII, p. 141; in German Studienausgabe IX, p. 411).
23 *Ibid.* My italics.
24 Why would there not be such an 'all the women'? Because of the Oedipus complex which places the mother under a prohibition? But the father also falls under a prohibition! Why at the point that we are at, should there be an 'all men' and not an 'all women'?
25 R. Blanché, *Les Structures intellectuelles*, Paris, Vrin, 1966, so: five years before Lacan's first attempts towards his formulae.
26 '*Non-universally*' (Blanché) becomes '*There exists*' (Lacan). We will come back to this point later on.
27 R Blanché, 'Sur le système des connecteurs interpropositionnels', in *Les cahiers pour l'analyse*, n°10, Paris, Le Seuil, hiver 1969, pp. 131–149. In the same issue of the same revue, there is Jacques Brunschwig's paper that has been paramount in Lacan's construction of his formulae.
28 In the syllogistic tradition the universal affirmative is named *a*, the particular affirmative *i*, the universal negative *e*, and the particular negative *o*. This notation will be followed in what follows.
29 This 'wavering' of the Lacanian formulae is precious, not for itself (the aesthetics of erudition) but for the liberty it gives with respect to written texts that too quickly become

canonical. Translation (Freud) and transcription (Lacan) often allow there to be found this wavering, which authorises the questions: 'Why did he say it like that rather than otherwise? How did he get to there?'

30 In other words, he already conceives as compatible (and not contradictory) the universal affirmative and the universal negative. This must soon be remembered when we enter into the logical square of the 'maximal' particular according to Brunschwig.

31 'Certainly there is indeed a reason to speak about indetermination, but 'indeterminate' is not a descriptive epitaph of 'number', it is rather an adverb modifying 'indicate'. We will not say that n designates an indeterminate number, but that it indicates numbers in an indeterminate manner'. 'What is a function?', in *Philosophical Writings of Gottlob Frege*, Oxford, Blackwell, 1993, p. 110.

32 Which Lacan was very fond of redoing on his own account because he also has in hand a domain peopled by individuals (the x of the formulae on the right) whom he claims, against the received opinion, escape from any collectivisation, any putting into a set that could be covered by an operator of the type $\forall$, exactly on the model of the famous 'sets that do not belong to themselves'.

33 On all these points, G. Le Gaufey, *L'incomplétude du symbolique*, Paris, EPEL, 1991, pp. 61-120.

34 G. Le Gaufey, 'Un événement logique: se découvrir mortel', *Les lettres de la SPF*, no. 9, SPF-Campagne-Première, 2003, pp. 135-146. On the web: www.legaufey.fr/106

35 Damourette et Pichon, *Des mots à Ia pensée*, tome I, Paris, Ed. D'Artrey, p. 138, section 115. Lacan had already given a substantial commentary on this around the sentence *Je crains qu'il ne vienne* (I am afraid that he will come), to the point of making of this *ne* the sign closest to the stating subject. Cf. 17 January 1962 in *Identification.*

36 J. Brunschwig, 'La proposition particulière et les preuves de non–concluance chez Aristote', *Cahiers pour L'analyse* no 10, Travaux du Cercle d'Epistémologie de l'ENS, Paris, Le Seuil, 1969, p. 326.

37 *Ibid.*, p. 22.

38 It will be remembered that the o-object is for its part also stripped in principle of any essence; otherwise, it would naturally fall under the concept.

39 D. Vernant, *Introduction à la logique standart*, Paris, Flammarion, 2001, p. 166.

40 In a very Russellian style, the sets that do not belong to themselves exist (they are legion), but that does not allow it to be thought for all that that they are grouped together, on the basis of this common feature, in a set of which each one would be an element.

41 Here one must get rid of the idea that they would not 'entirely' satisfy it (i.e. that a woman would never, as such, be 'entirely taken up into the phallic function', etc.) and that this would be the reason why Lacan would mark them with his 'not-all'.

42 J.-C. Milner, *Les penchants criminels de l'Europe démocratique*, Lagrasse, Verdier, 2003, pp. 17-20.

43 It is not at all a matter of making one the negation of the other but, on the contrary, the obstacle to the other.

44 Lacan, . . . *or Worse*, 8 December 1971.

45 Brunschwig, *op. cit.*, p. 7.

46 *Pas tous* (not all) and *pas tout* (not any) are equivalent here in the measure that when there is a regularly formed *tous*, in other words, a set in due and proper form, it is always possible to grasp any element whatsoever of it and to consider that 'for any' element and so on.

47 'The nothing that I am trying to get to hold up at this initial moment for you in the establishment of the subject is something different'. See above p. 31.

48 Hence the derived statements 'THE woman does not exist', 'The woman is not all', and so on, all formulations that gloss, each in its own way, the fact that the elements on the right do not form any set, any 'whole' from which one could pick out 'someone' or other.

49 That 'there is no metalanguage' is, in this respect, a harsh law, and if one still distinguishes something in it, it is those who momentarily forget this statement and who want clarity above all (since they are ready to pay from a cosmic viewpoint from which there is stated

the last distribution that they are aware of) and those who respect it at the price of rather quickly losing their way in it having wanted to remain faithful to the swirling function of the word.

50 Jacques Derrida used them no differently in his 'Le Facteur de la vérité' when he remarked that the letter, the object of so many sophisticated considerations on the part of Lacan, was found . . . between the legs of the chimney-piece (follow his look!).

51 Deixis is the name in the logical square for the elements that are ranked on the same side, what Lacan names then 'man' and 'woman'.

52 The apparent contradiction is not that difficult to understand. The formula comes from law, where it is asserted that 'the exception confirms the rule for all the cases non excepted'. This means that the law almost always anticipates exceptions and then gives a list of them. If any other exception is put forward in a particular case, it will be automatically discarded – because it does not belong to the list first given by the law. No mystery.

53 J. Lacan, *The Knowledge of the Psychoanalyst*, unpublished translation by Cormac Gallagher, 3 March 1972.

54 G. Le Gaufey, 'Belonging/Including', in *The Candidate*, New York, April 2015 (also: www.legaufey.fr/159). In this sense, there is indeed a set composed of the sets that belong to themselves, but there is only a *domain* composed of the sets that do not belong to themselves.

55 J. Lacan, 'L'étourdit', in *Scilicet* no. 4, Paris, Le Seuil, 1973, p. 15, or *Autres écrits*, Paris, Le Seuil, 2000, p. 458. I am giving here a triply corrected text. For the problem of establishing this passage and others, see the Addendum at the end of this chapter. More information in www.legaufey.fr/137 (only in French and Spanish), and for a general criticism of the first publication in French of *Le transfert*, see *Le transfert dans tous ses errata*, Paris, Epel, 1991 (www.epel-edition.com).

56 'I am combining [these two formulae] because the "there exists one" in question, by creating a limit to the "for any", is what affirms it or confirms it (which a proverb already objects to Aristotle's contradictory)'.

57 About these matters, see G. Le Gaufey, *L'incomplétude du symbolique*, Paris, EPEL, 1991.

3

SOME CLINICAL CONSEQUENCES OF THE LOGICAL DIFFERENCE BETWEEN THE SEXES

We have tried to follow as closely as possible the movements of the writing by which Lacan arrived at his formulae, in the hope of dissipating while doing so some stubborn obscurities, due in large measure to the interpretations that he was the first to make of them – among others, the one that sees in the exception, in $\exists x.\overline{\Phi x}$, the logical writing of the totemic father, of him who is supposed by definition to escape the phallic law valid for all, except for him. Taken in an uncritical way, this interpretation confuses a singular (there are never *x* totemic fathers per hoard, only one at a time) and a particular which, by definition, does not as such lay claim to singularity. At least in logic, where it is of overriding importance to distinguish between a particular proposition and a singular proposition which, for its part, implies one and only one individual, posing by this fact other problems apropos the existence of the element with respect to which it asserts something. Lacan, although giving the example of the totemic father, does not get involved in this confusion since he believes it appropriate to name this $\exists x.\overline{\Phi x}$ 'the-at-least-one-man' ('*l'hommoinzun*') and therefore leaves open the possibility that there are several of them capable of supporting this exception. By reducing the particular affirmative to a singular proposition, one is exposed inversely to missing out on the difficult status of the exception that this particular encircles because by bringing its extension down to just one individual, we may as well let the narcissism of each do as it will to reduce this exception to a 'self' (momentarily projected into the exceptional other) and, in this way, play half the fish caught by Lacan.

Likewise, a number of commentaries search in the not-all for some essence or other of femininity or for the enjoyment described as feminine, involving everything in a hopeless misunderstanding since what is at stake, from one end of the writings to the other, is deconstructing the possibility of a duality of essences in order to write a non-rapport.

We are nevertheless left with a serious problem on our hands. To have set aside from the outset any sense that might come from the appellations 'man' and 'woman' obliges us to give its place and its function to this bipartition. The initial *a priori*, that the formulae take over and deal with things in their own way but that they do not invent, comes down to distinguishing two sides, one for which it is affirmed that there does not exist an essence 'Woman',[1] and therefore not strictly a symbolic mapping out of this element, and the other where inversely we support the existence of an essence 'Man' which, for its part, develops a symbolic value of the element. At first sight, we are therefore dealing with an oppositional couple, and Milner might have been right to reduce the whole affair to the presence/absence of a distinctive trait.

The all and its strict bipartition

The refusal of the Freudian myth – 'there is no *all women*' – is not very solidly supported in this case. How conceive that 'Woman' does not accede to the pure symbol? One of the rare reasons that may here be invoked comes from the absence of the phallic trait, which would prevent the reduction of an individual to this single trait taking the place of symbol. Alas, a certain common sense, crossbred today with a structuralism decreed moreover to be superseded, has no longer any difficulty in seeing in the absence of a trait a decisive trait, which is how, in this precise case, it is mistaken.

To become aware of this, we must come up anew against the difficulty that punctuates this journey from the beginning: the impossible rapport between *difference* (which articulates relative terms) and the *quality* (which founds absolute, namely separate terms). If only the first, this man/woman difference, were at stake, it would be self-evident that the absence of a trait on one side would respond to the presence of the same trait on the other side and would therefore be valid as a trait qualifying Woman *as opposed* to Man. But let us now try to establish the quality that qualifies Man and the quality that qualifies Woman, without articulating them to one another from the outset. The absence of trait is no longer as quick to act as a reference point to subsume the diversity of (logical) individuals which do not find their place from the side of the presence of the trait, and we better understand Lacan's prudence in noting that in denying Man, one goes over to the Woman side but that in denying Woman nothing guarantees that one will go back to the Man side.[2] If, in effect, I deny the presence of a given trait, I get its absence, but if I deny its absence, how can I know that I am going to rediscover that very trait or a completely different one, or nothing at all? I would only rediscover it if I had given myself at the start a set composed exclusively of two subsets, 'Man' and 'Woman', in such a way that everything that is not on one side will be obligatory on the other. Lacan, as we have seen on several occasions, refuses this dualism, and this is the reason why the absence of phallic trait has no *complementary* value as compared to its presence, opening up by this very fact another space, liable to other rules.

Why does he reject this dualism? It would have been enough to adopt it to settle matters in the most classical way, by setting up the woman as the sexual object of the man and reciprocally, making both of them waltz with more or less happiness to the rowing-boat rhythm of the phallus. Now what creates an objection to this harmony is nothing but this little grain of sand, decisive for any self-respecting Freudian: *the drive does not entertain any natural and pre-established rapport to its object.* It indubitably aims at its own satisfaction, but the object that it requires to arrive at is, according to Freud, to be any one whatsoever:

> Experience of the cases that are considered abnormal has shown us that in the sexual instinct and the sexual object are merely soldered together – a fact which we have been in danger of overlooking in consequence of the uniformity of the normal picture, where the object appears to form part and parcel of the instinct. We are thus warned to loosen the bonds that exist in our thoughts between instinct and object. It seems probable that the sexual instinct is in the first instance independent of its object; nor is its origin likely to be due to its object attractions.[3]

Here is the turning point that Lacan, in his way, pursues beyond what Freud himself had been able to conclude from it. He was all the more inclined to do so in that there was spread out before him, under the colours of the most orthodox Freudianism, the enormity of the genital object that Freud himself had never produced. We have seen that if the drives *converge* on the primacy of the phallus, it is assuredly not under the heading of their object or thanks to it. The silent and naïve forging of the genital object in the French psychoanalysis of the 1950s *de facto* brought Freud's invention back into the mould of a normalising thought which no longer read in the aporias of the Oedipus complex any more than the matrix of a heterosexuality conceived as the therapeutic finality of analytic work. This genital object did not owe a whole lot to Freud, but a great deal to the French psychiatric tradition which, ever since Moreau de Tours, was based on the notion, at that time almost obvious, of the reproductive instinct (*instinct génésique*) which reduced human sexuality to procreation, as in the finest days of Christian moral theology since the 11th century.[4] Since an instinct guided the man towards the woman and reciprocally, it was enough to miss the Freudian step that uncoupled *Trieb* and *Object* to fall straight onto this genital object. Every deviation with respect to this instinct allowed the new concept of 'perversion' to be thought out with the musty smell of unhealthy pathology that accompanied this nosographical term. To slip up on this point, to hold men and women to be naturally *complementary*, came back therefore to abandoning psychoanalysis to psychology which, under the cover of 'the science of man', was in the process of acquiring its academic dignity and already sought to establish on the Freudian terrain a clinic suitable to give some lustre to a psychopathology wanting to distinguish itself from psychiatry. One can imagine why Lacan was intent on fighting against this current and for that reason to set up a fundamental disequilibrium in the inevitable bipartition of the human being.

He found himself, in effect, warned by the fact that the same logical gesture serves to establish a strict duality between the sexes (even if it entails refining it subsequently in ambiguous cases), and to partition living beings into normal and pathological (with the same innumerable border problems). In both cases, one is silently presupposing a world, a closed well circumscribed given that one then divides in a clairvoyant way into two opposed and complementary parts, with the then unavoidable consequence that being absent from one side equals being present on the other. Inversely, by becoming attentive to the mutual support lent by a strict bipartition of one class into two subclasses and the universal which, thanks to its 'for-all', is able to find in each of these subclasses what is not in the other, one can better divine how the logical regulation of the sexes insofar as they are supposed to be substantially two and the sovereign hold of the universal in the operation of the concept are two sides of the same coin. Sex and logic have indeed a shared interest, at least in their way of being deceptive (*d'en imposer*) in counting up to two.

The merit of the formulae of sexuation comes down, first of all, to not treating separately these two aspects of the same question and operating on the universal so that, by making it trip up at the right place, to deconstruct the sexually opposed couple which, in a first phase, served to pose it. The whole trick depends on ensuring that this equilibrium does not generate any symmetry, that the trait present on the left (which grounds the all) and the absence of trait on the right (which requires a not-all) do not share any already circumscribed space. Within a completely different horizon, when rewriting the Saussurian algorithm of the sign to accommodate it to his preoccupations, we remember that Lacan was careful to leave entirely to one side the band encircling signifier and signified, both separated by the bar.[5] It is the same here: one must go to the trouble of exploding the circle, not drawn, to be sure, but oh how easily thought, that could surround the formulae and bring them back to an inner articulation of one and the same space, that of the phallic function insofar as it would be numerically restricted.

From the universal to the concept

To get to the point of taking one's distance vis-à-vis so natural a suggestion, which tends to enclose a field once it has been posed, it would be well to return to the reasons that fortify Lacan in his struggle against the universal affirmative proposition, in a clear way since at least 1962. Why does he insist that at the level of the universal negative, and in accordance with the example that he takes of the universal affirmative 'all traits are vertical', there should be stated, not 'all traits are not vertical' but 'there is no trait (which is not vertical)'? Why privilege the nothing where Aristotle, Apuleius, and Kant (among so many others!) saw only a plurality of subjects denying the predicate of the universal affirmative? We have to look hard to encounter some clear affirmation on this point. On 7 March 1962, nevertheless, he puts forward the following:

> In the first disc of the circle [in other words the top right quadrangle, the universal negative] it is a matter of preserving the rights of the nothing, on top, because it is what creates below the perhaps, namely, the possibility. Far

> from being able to say as an axiom – and this is the stupefying error of the whole abstract deduction of the transcendental – far from being able to say that anything real is possible, it is only starting from the not possible that the real takes its place. What the subject is looking for is this real qua precisely not possible; it is the exception.

We have been able to see that such a decision only found its consistency much later in Lacan by basing itself on the *maximal* particular, but from 17 January of this same year, from the bringing into operation of different logical propositions on the basis of a universal negative affirming 'there is no man who does not lie,[6] he comes to ask the question, 'What interest do we have in using a system like this?' His response is worth quoting at length:

> What we contribute to renew the question is the following: I am saying that Freud promulgates, puts forward the following formula: the father is God or every father is God. There results, if we maintain this proposition at the universal level: there is no other father but God, which on the other hand as regards existence is in Freudian reflection rather *aufgehoben*, rather suspect, indeed radically in doubt. What is involved is that the order of function that we are introducing with the name of the father is this something which, at the same time, has its universal value, but which leaves to you, to the other, the task of determining whether there is or not a father of this stature. If none exists, it is still true that the father is God, simply the father is only confirmed by the empty sector of the dial . . . it is precisely these two sectors . . . which gives their full import to what we can state as universal affirmation.

What limits the range of the universal affirmative in Lacan's eyes is therefore double: not alone does it find itself denied by the particular affirmative which supports the existence of exceptions, but by reason of this choice of the maximal particular, the universal affirmative agrees with the universal negative (they are conjointly true or false) while this latter no longer takes account of any subject – this is the novelty. We have here, all of a sudden, a handling of the universal that right away goes beyond the sexual question since the central concept produced at that time by Lacan – the name-of-the-father – is for its part also liable to the same economy, as we have just read: its truth is not brought into play at the simple level of the particulars (yes, there are some of them that verify this statement, and others not), but it tolerates very well the total absence of realisation. Here is the nothing whose 'rights it is a matter of preserving' and which explodes Pierce's well-circled quadrangle to which people too often reduce Lacan's formulae (it is true that, here also, he was the first to do it).

It is a matter of hammering in at every level that the Other is not one, that what is valid for the big-Other-treasury-of-signifiers is valid for the sex-Other, that no *heteros* encloses the *allos*, that no *alter* subsumes the *alius*, that man and woman are not aliquot parts in sex but indeed aliquant; that the sets that do not belong to themselves are not to be accounted for like those that belong to themselves, and so forth. The incompleteness which already gave its make-up to the Lacan style of symbolic is indispensable in the question of sex once it is a matter of writing its internal logic to put to work this symbolic by which are announced the universal propositions which allow being predicated a certain number of individuals, to be fabricated a knowledge on the different postures with respect to phallic enjoyment. But this incompleteness, henceforth taken up again in the form of logical formulae which in detailing its functions, also involves a different positioning vis-à-vis the theory that psychoanalysis requires. How do these formulae take umbrage at the classical handling of the concept? How do they come to cut across this other fateful couple, theory/practice?

The two types of logical contrariety

To understand this, we must allow ourselves to return for the last time to the double acceptation of the particular, maximal and minimal. That Aristotle should have judged it right to set one of them aside to better settle the question which concerned him, and that via Apuleius and some others this decision should have weighed heavily on the history of logic, all that has not got rid of the problem that is at once logical, language-dependent, and sexual since it depends on the ambiguity of the opposition of contraries at the level of universals, which determines the double value of the particular: sometimes the contraries are presented like the two extremes of the same genus (from the one to the other, there is a continuity), and sometimes they are incarnated in terms which cannot tolerate being united and mutually exclude one another (between the two there is a separation).

How differentiate with complete clarity contrariety by contrast and contrariety by incompatibility? There is little chance that their negation will produce the same result! And we have been able to see that this question is par excellence the one posed by the sexes, which sometimes oppose one another without excluding one another, reciprocally complement one another, and sometimes are excluded one from the other, incarnating in their own way the double value of the *or*, sometimes inclusive and sometimes exclusive (respectively, *vel* and *aut* in Latin). But the approach through the particulars presents, first of all, the interest of showing us how the logical square which seems to inspire respect by its perfect order is itself defective.

What differences can one legitimately conceive between the particular affirmative ($\exists x.\overline{\Phi x}$) and the particular negative ($\overline{\forall x}.\Phi x$)? For the first, the tongue comes to our help by saying 'some' and for the second Lacan takes over an expression of Aristotle and raises it to a neologism with his 'not-all'; on one hand, an affirmation of existence – yes, there are indeed at least some – and, on the other hand, a restriction – some, yes, but not all. A precious detail . . . for the logician much more than for the speaker, who has most often perfectly well interpreted *some* in its restrictive value with respect to the all. If I learn that 'some' passengers have lost their lives in an air crash, I will not for a single moment imagine that all having been lost, I am informed that at least some have been. Brunschwig's 'maximal' sense is the first that the tongue promotes, and far from being complex (the union of the partitive and of the restrictive), it appears there as the most simple term: the partitive is from the start a restrictive, and if one wants it not to be so, if one leans, like the logicians towards the minimal sense of the particular, then and then only is it appropriate to go against the tongue by specifying what is not self-evident, namely that 'some, because all', that the particular affirmative is in this case only a partial instantiation of a universal truth (in the universe of the chosen discourse, the scientific one par excellence which, in its search for universal truths, is only interested in minimal particulars). Leibnitz himself worked hard at finding a distinction between the restrictive *some* and the indeterminate *some*, when the Venn diagrams[7] proved, for their part, to be incapable of representing separately the two types of particulars, which in logic earns them the qualification of 'troublesome propositions' in the measure that the senses that they distinguish refer to affirmative and negative universals that are sometimes contradictory and sometimes equivalent.

The logical square, in effect, associates each particular to its universal according to quality: the affirmatives to the left, the negatives to the right. Besides, in both cases of the particular (maximal and minimal), a relation of contradiction is maintained between each universal and its opposite particular according to quality: the particular affirmative denies the universal negative, and the particular negative denies the universal affirmative. The double sense of contrariety, that was difficult to read at the level of two universals, is transparent then in their negation in the measure that the tongue only offers a single word for the existential particular affirmative and the restrictive particular negative: some. By choosing the minimal sense, Aristotle and the logical tradition privileged the 'some' of the particular affirmative which the denies the 'null' of the universal negative, without any restrictive nuance, and leaves the field free to the *dictum de omni*, to the fact that this *some* is implied by the universal affirmative: 'some because all'. By only coming second, the restrictive negative particular, the one obtained by denying the universal affirmative, loses a lot by also using *some* since, to remove the equivocation of this supposedly simple element, we have to add 'some but not all', in other words the restriction which qualifies this position in the maximal version.

Lacan for his part remains within the limits of the classical logical square (at no time does he take on board the 'logical hexagon' proposed by R. Blanché in his *Structures intellectuelles*), but he inverts its values. Under its apparent symmetry, the Aristotelian logical square inclined to the left by favouring the particular affirmative, as much by the fact of its agreement with the universal affirmative as by its ontological weight resulting from its contradiction with the universal negative; that of Lacan inclines, for its part, to the right by giving priority to the not-all, to the particular negative, to the point that the particular affirmative, the $\exists x.\overline{\Phi x}$ only manages to be written as a negation of the universal negative and not as a part of the universal affirmative, since it contradicts it. Blanché himself, in tackling the same logical square, explicitly takes into account the difficulty in conceiving the particular affirmative at first as the negation of the universal negative: 'The only true opposites, the remark has been made more than once, are those that are mutually exclusive, namely the contraries and the contradictories. That is why, in the logical square itself, the construction of the fourth position *i* (the particular affirmative) with the negation has something indirect and forced about it'.[8] The fact that this particular affirmative produced in this way enters into contradiction with the universal affirmative ($\forall x.\Phi x$) is therefore not first (as a number of commentaries try to establish in interpreting from the start this particular as an exception to the rule of the universal) but results from the prior affirmation of the not-all (first stage in the construction of the particulars of the square of the formulae of sexuation) since, by denying the universal affirmative, this particular negative leaves the field free to the $\overline{\exists x}.\Phi x$ of the particular affirmative (it will be remembered that they are equivalent, that they are therefore true or false conjointly).

By privileging, with his 'not-all', the restrictive aspect of the particular negative which has kept in check the universal affirmative as well as the negative, Lacan at once agrees with the tongue and empties the universal of its residual ontology. In the classical Aristotelian acceptation, 'all men' possessed indeed some existence, supported as it was by this particular existential which had lent it assistance by offering it the shelter of a 'some' in harmony with it. With the Lacan version of the logical square, we are finished with that: 'all men' becomes a strictly symbolic element on which it is, of course, permitted to predicate ($\forall x.\Phi x$) but whose existence nothing assures for the moment. The universal negative makes the thing still more explicit since in it we allow ourselves to predicate in the absence of a subject: $\overline{\exists x}.\overline{\Phi x}$.

The particular existentials, affirmative and negative, are therefore no longer the partial instantiations of universal truths. Quite the contrary, they are only valid by wrong-footing it, by objecting to the universality that they reject by common disagreement. To suppose that all say yes ($\forall x.\Phi x$) and that there are none who say no ($\overline{\exists x}.\overline{\Phi x}$), those who say no ($\exists x.\overline{\Phi x}$), and those who say yes ($\overline{\forall x}.\Phi x$) cock a double snoot at the statements that claim to govern them.

The consistency of analytic knowledge

This logical arrangement explained in this way creates a new epistemological situation, and the degree to which it suits psychoanalytic knowledge remains to be appreciated, inasmuch as it also presents a very singular *consistency*. First, some remarks to approach the latter, impossible to pinpoint using a local observation in the measure that it involves a global property.

After a century of proliferation, one can affirm that this knowledge is cumulative to an extraordinarily small degree. Who could claim to have yet added a stone to the Freudian edifice? The men and women who have worked in this field (today they are almost legion) may be accepted as having built on Freudian foundations – otherwise, the adjective would escape them – but their developments scarcely amount to adding to the Freudian corpus to form a new homogeneous whole. Disparity remains essential for the comprehension of their work, and if Freud lends to each of them more or less of his knowledge[9] (just as everyone is very careful to anchor in the Freudian text the essential of his own inventions), the respect for the heterogeneity of the corpus remains the condition for an attentive reading of the different authors. This is why psychoanalysis is resolutely not a science since, in this field, if the historian knows how to render to Caesar what belonged to Caesar, the manuals which serve to transmit established knowledge have no need to scrupulously respect the diversity of contributors.

Each generation of analysts must in this way 'learn its lessons' by reading Freud, most often through the spectacles of some lineage of commentators. A major part of analytic literature is thus composed of exercises in learning the Freudian language (Lacanian, Kleinian, Bionian, etc.), which have scarcely any ambition to innovate but serve as a step at the entrance of the corporation. No criticism in this remark which is only there to underline the style of the acquisition of a knowledge of undeniable richness in texts to be shared and of a no less certain poverty in experiences with which to sympathise. On this last point, each one only refers to him- or herself and to his or her presuppositions regarding the others around, a great difference to the scientific researcher who has almost more facilities for sharing his experiences than his theories.

Faced with this particularity, perilous for the transmission of their practice, analysts have rather quickly reacted along two different and even divergent paths, each one seeking nevertheless to constitute a homogeneous field, apt to subsume the diversity of authors and situations that it claims to include: on one hand, the academic path, which offers to psychoanalysis the consistency of a higher education knowledge with its degrees, with its titulars, its diplomas, and its regularly renewed audience and, on the other, rather relegated in institutes and other schools despite its frankly medical model, a clinic is put in place which, saddled without any other form of procedure with the adjective *psychoanalytic*, aspires to what academic knowledge does not even lay claim to: to transmit the very core of analytic experience, beyond theoretical diversities held to be irreducible and from that to install the psychoanalyst in his operational legitimacy.

Such a clinic nevertheless suffers, at first sight, from a constitutive defect. The one that medicine invented presents itself on a sort of irreducible tripod in which the natural signs of illness offer themselves (anyway, almost! I am not forgetting that it is very often necessary to circumscribe them, which has nothing neutral about it, but there is no question of fabricating them) to a double look: the partly naïve one of the pupil desiring to establish the difference between his book learning and the reality of illness and the learned and pragmatic one of the experienced clinician of the fundamental equivocation of signs held to be pathological. Psychoanalysis, for its part, obliged as it is to refuse any third party in its arrangements, cannot produce any clinical sign as a natural sign, observable by anyone whomsoever lay or professional. How could a clinic be constituted while being incapable of offering to the signs that it promotes the space in which they might be unfolded without any other artifice?

On the vignette-style case

This crucial (and constitutive) deficiency has led to a terribly ambiguous conception of the *case*. Since it has from all time had its Freudian letters patent of nobility, many pretend not to see any problem in it: If Freud did it, why should we not do it, we who want to be Freudians? Here, the etymology of the word *author* can help, because indeed it is 'authority' that is at stake. When Freud wrote some of the different cases that punctuate his work, he based himself on a historicity of events of which he gives more or less an account, inviting us by this very fact to swallow his version of the facts.[10] Can one imagine a clinical tutor who would consider as sufficient to 'recount' the signs that the student should be able to identify in the perceptual magma that awaits him in his medical practice? Magisterial lectures overflow with these descriptions of signs, accompanied by their rational explanations! What is expected, on the contrary, from a clinic worthy of the name, is that an undiscovered sign might find its place in the theoretical knowledge which integrates it into the heart of a rational texture. The clinic appears in this sense as the locus of a deictics charged with making the liaison between a fragment of theoretical knowledge, where the sign is described in its rational and relational complexity, and the *hic et nunc* of a sign received and perceived in the opacity of its presence.

Nothing of the kind in what concerns the account of a psychoanalytic case, where one is bound to believe the one who recounts it. Just as much as if it were a master, otherwise . . . the case runs the risk of being forgotten before even having touched existence. Hence the paradox: the psychoanalytic clinic is only sustained by magisterial cases, and leaves in the shadows of its immense befuddled literature the swarm of clinical accounts. Even Lacan, who is so often accused of not having spoken about 'his cases', will have left behind him enough to construct a certain number, the man of the fresh brains, Joyce, Lucie Tower, without forgetting his entry into psychoanalysis, Marguerite Anzieu, Aimée. The fact that they have in the main been constructed by his pupils more than by himself does not change the deal: they hold their authority, first of all, from his first footprint.

This style of transmission of the case is evidently not the prerogative of psychoanalysis. Psychiatry itself has produced throughout its short history celebrated cases,[11] which have served as a touchstone for theoretical confrontations in this field. And one might just as well launch oneself here into a detailed study of moral or religious casuistry to discover the same phenomenon. Nevertheless, people do not for all that speak there about 'clinic': they are content to start from a common narrative, to open up the range of possible interpretations. What therefore in our day is called 'clinical' in psychoanalysis?

If one keeps to one side the flood of psychopathological publications, who think they depend on the clinic because they treat of entities that are themselves held to be clinical (hysteria, phobia, infantile psychosis, negative transference, etc.), there remains a swarm of little texts, disseminated in general in articles or books that can be differently described but which all take a case into account, in a few lines or a few pages (maximum). This has been called for 30 or so years, no more, 'clinical vignettes', and the success of appellation has been such that it has passed without difficulty into English ('clinical vignette'), as well as Spanish (*viñetas clínicas*).

The word *vignette* appeared at first in the form of *vigneture* (French), to designate ornaments in the shape of a grapevine leaf that framed medieval miniatures. But when typography got involved in it, it took over the word to signify 'the ornamental motif printed on top of the first page of a book or a chapter, then to any position on the page'.[12] From then on, the word, without changing its first sense, invaded multiple sectors of daily life: playing cards, commercial labels, fiscal stamps (the *vignette automobile* and others),[13] without neglecting its first love: *cul-de-lampes*. It is even charged already with a stereotyped sense with the expression '*faire vignette*' towards the end of the 19th century.[14]

Whatever the difference of workmanship in these vignettes that ornament, decorate, garland, enhance, embellish, adorn remarks that one fears lack some flesh, it is remarkable that they all accomplish the same task, which moreover justifies their appellation: *to illustrate*, by a demonstrative example, some statement that is too arid and because of this is qualified as 'theoretical'. Rather than falling back on what is very often caricatural in this literature, I am choosing here in something I have recently read a text of some amplitude, which sets out describe the course of a treatment in a dozen or so pages.[15] After a very detailed account, approaching the conclusion, we read the following:

> It thus appears to me that, in the Winnicottian perspective which I hold to, the phobic manifestations described here can be completely understood as so many means Pauline used to protect herself against this threat of a collapse, 'a danger that one looks for in the future even though it took place in the past'.

I would not dream here either of criticising a reference to Winnicott rather than to some other author or of casting doubt on the pertinence, relative to the case, of this theoretical and practical support taken by the analyst throughout this treatment. What is important to me on the contrary is the 'can be completely understood' which states in the apparently prudent style of possibility, a link of implication between the Winnicottian thesis of the fear of collapse in phobias because of a melancholic kernel inherited from this time before the ego/non-ego differentiation[16] and the tribulations of the aforenamed Pauline. This link, present throughout the text, is reaffirmed in the summary:

> In a Winnicottian perspective, the course of the treatment has, in fact, allowed there to be progressively highlighted a defensive organisation against a subjective collapse of a melancholic type. The particular affirmative – Pauline and the account of her undoubted and romantic existence – does indeed fall, even if it is *grosso modo*, into the abstract category that every reader of Winnicott knows, at least in its major lines; but why produce a harmony of this kind between a case and what it is supposed to depend on to respond to a certain idea of the clinic according to which knowledge is congruent to the reality that it describes? In a first phase, this appears so obvious, so simple, that it is not easy to see the bundle of hypotheses that accompany this vision.

If I produce a concept, it is indeed in effect with the idea that a certain number of objects and/or situations *correspond* to its definition, and that therefore the links that it entertains with its colleagues, the other concepts, are so many directions for research proposed to my study. There is no fault to be found in this; most knowledge, including scientific, go along with this. Now a concept is like a universal in that it claims to state something that is valid for *all the individuals* who 'fall' under it. It intends to subsume them to make itself the bearer of a truth which, belonging to each one, is valid for all, and allows this plurality to be treated as a unity, liable to relations up to then unexpected with other unities of the same order.

Nevertheless, our prior logical journey has shown that such an implication of the universal towards its particular only takes up the minimal particular and that this type of logical functioning cannot claim to be the only rigorous one; the maximal can just as well do so, even though it objects to the universal of the same quality (and what is more, to the other as well). It then becomes possible to free oneself a little from the intimidation with which a certain rationality intends to reduce every use of the concept to the subsuming of positive occurrences, and to envisage the rapport of the concept with every existence, whatever it may be, in an eminently contradictory way: no longer a rapport of congruence but of active refusal. *The trait that the object, the situation or the individual presents, and which allows them to be ranged under a particular concept, is in effect not of the same nature as the trait present in the concept.*[17] This point, almost illegible in the minimal particular, explodes in the maximal. To take a trivial example, if 'all say yes' ($\forall x.\Phi x$), to affirm that 'there exist some who do not say yes' ($\exists x.\overline{\Phi x}$), right away places these some in an existence that gives first place to the presence of the symbolic trait since I take them into account even when they do not flaunt it. In affirming existences that do not fall under the concept, I give precedence to existence, and in so doing, without in any way attacking the conceptual order itself, I offer it, on the contrary, a possibility of consisting otherwise than as the map of a country that is already there, otherwise then as a map that might offer me, to scale and with a great economy of effort, an opportunity for me to locate myself, thanks to a cohort of organised signs, in the overcomplicated and diverse world of my perceptions.

To give precedence to one or other of the two types of particular does not depend therefore simply on a technical choice, as Aristotle's decision might be thought to be, but involves almost diametrically opposed perspectives in the way of making a knowledge operate relative to the experiences that it frames. The promotion of the 'polemical fact' in Bachelard's epistemology is characteristic of a dominance of the maximal particular in the search for the experiment that is going to bring a contradiction to a scientific law received up to then, even though the teaching and the transmission of this very law will be inscribed, without having any need to specify it, in the framework of the minimal particular. However exclusive they may be to one another, neither of these two opinions can claim to lay down the law and to reign alone, *without our being able moreover to articulate them rationally with one another* (a sort of logical premonition of 'There is no [sexual] rapport'). There is here a hiatus that gives rise to two often enemy spiritual families, often deaf to one another, something William James took account of in the following way:

> The strife of these two kinds of mental temper will, I think, always be seen in philosophy. Some men will keep insisting on the reason, the atonement that lies at the heart of things, and *in conformity* with what we can act; others, on the opacity of brute fact that we must react *against*.[18]

For one side, conceptual architecture, first of all, expresses the order of the world. For the others, first of all, it misses it, and from this very missing, the object shines forth and is anchored in existence: 'Is there a concept of a footstep arriving in the dark?', asks Yves Bonnefoy,[19] '[O]f the fall of a stone in the undergrowth, of the impression made by an empty house? Of course not. *Nothing of the real has been kept except what preserves our peace*'. I have no intention here of reconciling these two approaches but, on the contrary, of marking the divergent paths that they open up in the 'psychoanalytic clinic'.

The clinical vignette and its order

The clinical vignette was born in the crucible of the minimal particular by reason of its belief in conformity (up to that, nothing serious), but it very quickly surrounded this exercise with a naivety that makes it ignore the limits of its relevance and inflates it then with a false scientific and moral rigour which tends to exclude it from the very clinic that it lays claim to. For, by wanting to only illustrate, it is prevented and forbidden from criticising so that the theoretical fragment taken as a reference, whatever may be its breadth, emerges from it with a fearsome reality coefficient.

Since there are existences – those of which an account is being given – that are organised more or less according to the conceptual scaffolding invoked, then the latter is not simply a symbolic construction, a bundle of articulated meanings, but the exact reflection of the workings of the real world! The Platonic cave, always lying in wait for a thought that is organising itself, surreptitiously regains the upper hand once one leaves the field free to the idea according to which existences are above all shadows taken from Ideas. Add up the clinical vignettes, and you will no longer be able to get out of a realism which erects the chosen theory into a superego with a voracity that goes beyond its knowledge: immense, pernickety, despotic – protective.

In this way, the clinical vignette triumphs in what Thomas S. Khun was able to call the 'normal' periods and surroundings of psychoanalysis, those in which a paradigm has acquired such power in a given milieu that to question it as regards its own consistency is ruled out. It both reigns and governs since, fully occupied with organising a supposed bric-a-brac, it clothes itself with a legitimacy that affects naturalness by basing itself on common sense: One cannot use a tool and at the same time make it, no? This is the obligated riposte of all established powers: they take all sorts of trouble to dominate the world for its own greater good, and people want them in addition, at the same time, to be transformed, even be soft-sawdered! A kind of indignation often disturbs the evocation of such perspectives, which are to be expected from irresponsible people.

Since paradigms do not show themselves openly, it is moreover necessary that the power in place should produce, or at least authorise, a vulgate of this knowledge that serves as reference; to reinvigorate from time to time its major outlines; in a more hidden way, it and it alone should be recognised as having access to alterations of the fundamental pattern, because it is from it that all life comes. This textual and theoretical model that focuses the collectivity must therefore be at once living and fixed, life-giving and organising, present and in reserve. Its power has the responsibility to get to the bottom of the diversity of the real since, as an interpretative grill, the vocation of this model is to deal with the variety of situations, but – outside the official retoucher – no one is authorised to question it because then there would be a risk that the boxes of the grill would begin to operate in an anarchic fashion and run the risk of invalidating the interpretations already given and would run the risk finally of revealing the flaws of this prestigious construction.

The vignette is therefore not a little ornament that is added on to make things look true, and which one could well do without. It shares in a general economy which joins to an unacknowledged philosophical realism a centralised political order, the (local) holder of the legitimacy of the founding text. It promises a semiotics in which the sign is at its foundation an index of the real. It is certainly the reason why we have been able to see such an insistence, among certain Lacanians who are great users of clinical vignettes, on the 'anchoring points' mentioned by Lacan who, in one or other session of his Seminar on *The Psychoses*, engages himself to give 'the minimum number of fundamental points of attachment between the signifier and the signified necessary for a human being to be called normal and which, when they are not established, or when they give way, produce the psychotic'.[20] Subsequently, he hardly ever mentions these very risky anchoring points, but it was a godsend for the clinical vignettes, still to come at the time, which are based on this conviction that there are, all the same, a minimal number unmistakable signs. Thus, one can read, in number 52 of the journal *La Cause freudienne*,

> Lacan posed that there is in the experience of an analysis an anchoring point, that of the traversing of the phantasy, that it is a matter of demonstrating one by one in accordance with a regular procedure. If subsequently he did investigate the beyond of this anchoring point, it nevertheless remains that he set up from 1967 on the examination of analytic experience, of its results and of its conclusion, at the heart of the analytic community, forcing it to say each time, case by case, what a psychoanalysis is.[21]

The vignette confines us to a determined type of relationship to the text since the relations of authority between the two are such that the victor is known in advance. It being ruled out that one should brandish a case that would make up a proof by direct observation, just imagine the number of pages needed to establish one that would try to contradict . . . let us say Lacan's statement according to which 'there is no sexual *rapport*' or Freud's statement 'every dream is a wish fulfillment'. With this complication, fatal on the Freudian terrain mined by denegation: whoever wants to prove too much . . .

This order in which the vignette is inscribed would not call for so much criticism if it did not go against, not alone a certain number of theses present in the theoretical corpus we are illustrating but even its most immediate aims. At first sight, the vignette, in effect, offers, in narrative mode and through a language unaffected in the best cases, individuals and events towards which our interest is naturally drawn. In fact, the first lines of a well-written vignette are rather agreeable to read and give the feeling of opening a window in a stuffy room. But this impression invariably turns sour, and the Paulines, the Bernards, the Cs, and the Ps rather quickly become strange ectoplasms; once their use has been divined, they become really needy, as white as Gilles rolled in flour, with their big red clowns' noses. The singularity that they seemed to have as a mission to defend against the steam roller of a faceless theory is reduced to the little finger on the seam of the trousers supposed to accompany the vibrant and sonorous 'Present!' that responds to the roll call in a barrack room. The living flesh expected blanches by showing itself so submissive, and it is still worse when the proliferation of details thickens without anyone ever making any speculative difficulty for the interpretation which, in the end, is going to imprison them.

One might nevertheless think that we are dealing with a complex and varied rhetorical form, so developed in Freudian literature for almost a century that it would be excessive to reduce it to such a servile function. People still praise the little spontaneous writings of a Ferenczi, the clinical richness of a Klein. But the promotion of the clinical vignette is more recent and denotes something other than the Freudian appeal to the case: it responds to the fixation of the Lacanian paradigm and its setting up as a battery in a collectivity engaged in acquiring a professional mastery and of structuring itself on this foundation. Nevertheless, what is most important, beyond its sociological function in the analytic milieu, is that the clinical vignette should be based in such a massive and unsuspected way on the minimal particular because, from that, an imperious logic determines how it is used and predisposes it to miss out on some of Lacan's fundamental intuitions regarding the sexes and the standing of analytic knowledge in the clinic of that name.

'There is no sexual *rapport*' marks a disparity between the sexes such that, far from reducing sexual difference, it amplifies it to the point of making them incommensurable; now this is only obtained by basing oneself from the start on the maximal particular, which invalidates the universal affirmative, which therefore right away puts a spoke in the wheel of the case which would be content to illustrate the veracity of a theoretical statement. If a particular affirmative happens, in effect, in the supposed naivety of its existence, to confirm the universality of a concept (or of a conceptual concatenation), and by so doing puts in place a minimal particular, good-bye to the not-all! It will no longer have any chance of emerging, except emptied of its sense or charged with the misunderstanding which would make of it the brand of a Woman essence – for one does not navigate without inconsequence between the logical squares.

The realism that the vignette insidiously develops leads, for its part, to more direct and more visible consequences as regards the medicalisation of analytic knowledge. The apparent promotion of the clinical point of view, with its well-advertised distrust of theory, is in this regard mistaken: since the account that is given derives its power from its value as a direct index, from its way of pointing towards a reality as rigidly as a Kripke-style index, the theory becomes a reservoir of names, a heap of terms, a toolbox. All of a sudden, its internal architecture, its possible contradictions, uncertainties, or bragging no longer have any status, and practically do not exist. The theoretical statements are positive or do not exist. This obviously silent reduction withdraws them from the field of polemics emptied by this of its substance and produces a sort of irenicism of the vignette, which has nothing fortuitous about it since any *internal* debate relative to the consistency of the paradigm is ruled out – only the modalities of its application to the case are open for discussion. This same irenicism nevertheless reverses into warlike passion if someone tries to introduce, in however small a way, a paradigm foreign to it, which in that case is rather considered of as anything more than stupidity, ignorance, or bad faith, nothing that is worth discussing. In this way, the vignette leaves a free hand to the *practitioners* who intend to exercise their art in connecting a knowledge (constructed by others) and a nature (that God, or Evolution, or society have made such in its profuse pathology). Now they have become doctors of the soul, psychotherapists.

Here, I have stressed the trait to separate out one of the axes between two heterogeneous, logically incompatible positions. It is self-evident that things are more complex, more overlapping, in part because analysts, as practitioners, are not – here we are hoping! – so consequent, do not set up rigor as such a constant ideal, and know how to let go of it . . . at the right time. I maintain that we are not continuously moving from one logical square to the other; but nothing stops people from doing so . . . in a discontinuous way! Thus, anyone who chances a vignette is not *ipso facto* obliged to swallow all its deviations, and it can happen that someone momentarily follows this path without becoming too bogged down and hung up on its underlying logic.[22] But it is rare.

Outline of a maximal clinic

It now remains to see some clinical consequences of the maximal particular, when the affirmations of existence effectuated at the level of particulars each wrong-foot the two universals, the affirmative as well as the negative. The existents constitute an *exception* – that is their status – without our rushing into thinking that because of this they are rare as compared to the all (since the all of the maximal universal does not imply any existence at its level and the universal negative is empty). We must therefore now come to think of the *existence* of the exception as a *qualitative* phenomenon, without unduly basing ourselves on the quantitative which, by isolating a minimal percentage of individuals over against a majority put into the position of quasi-universality, would surreptitiously draw from it the notion of exception.

Having posed the very terms of the problem, Lacan proposed a solution by producing the asymptote of the hyperbola as an example of exception able to serve as a foundation. I had in this very book the opportunity to criticise this solution which singularises the exception too much and tends to maximise the existence of the elements of all (the infinity of the points of the curve) and to minimise the exception value (the zero, corresponding to the ordinate axis). The advantage of the figuration – the curve does indeed give the impression of being 'based' on its asymptote – is reversed in the respective ontological weights of the regular values of the curve and of the zero of the abscissa of the asymptote, which itself reproduces the exception to singularity. This figurative support does not therefore suffice to express the fact of the plural exception on the left of the formulae (it totally misses the *at-least-one*, *l'hommoinzun*) or its absence on the right; in this, Lacan does not do justice to the discovery in his writings, and his mathematical commentary falls short of his logical audacity.[23]

In fact, we may begin to have a presentiment that no example will allow us to grasp status of the exception that Lacan produces in his formulae for this exception cannot be reduced to one or several cases which would be excepted from the universal affirmative, leaving it amputated as it were from these elements which contradict it. This very set-oriented or Eulerian comprehension considers the universal as a sort of general rule capable of undergoing some exceptions without ceasing for all to govern the majority of cases. We too quickly find ourselves with this kind of vision in the quantitative considerations which treat the universal and the particular on the same existential footing and make of the exception nothing other than a minority derogating from the common law. Now this silent deduction is no longer appropriate once there has been launched the Lacan-style 'not-all', which goes well beyond the Brunschwig style of maximal particular by reason of its treatment of the affirmation of existence (reduced to particular propositions), even though universals are totally deprived of it.

If these short logico-ontological considerations appear abstruse, we can here have recourse to the elementary logical rule of *modus ponens*, which brings to light the same dislocation by postulating that if the implication 'if A therefore B' is true, and nothing more . . . nothing follows from it. However true this statement may be, it will not bring about any consequences unless someone is in a position to affirm that 'it is true that A', in which case the previously mentioned implication unfolds its truth, and affirms then, and only then, that B is true. As long as no existence is affirmed from the point of view of the antecedent, from the point of view of A, the implication remains inert. It conveys a certain knowledge by describing the constraining relations between two terms, two propositions, two concepts, but as long as the antecedent is not realised, this knowledge remains ineffective.

What then is the mode of subsistence of such an implication *before* some existential or other comes to affirm of one of these elements that it is (or is not) the case? This question, or others in the same vein, crisscrossed the first steps of the new formal logic. In Frege, for example, it is found in the form of the fundamental opposition between 'objects' and 'functions'. A function is a sort of proposition which always presents (by definition) an empty place, which must be occupied by an object for the aforesaid function to be activated and gives birth to a meaning, which itself possesses (or not) a reference, and at the same time a truth value. As long as it is not endowed with any object, the function presents a very curious level of existence. One cannot really say that it belongs to this world in which we live. Objects, from their point of view, do not present any internal lack (by definition), and quietly wait until a function wants to engage with them so that they can participate in a knowledge. They exist, without for all that 'being' in the sense that Quine was able to detach by his formula according to which 'to be, is to be the value of a variable': as long as an object is not possessed by a function under the heading of variable, the question of its being is not even posed: its existence, curiously, takes precedence over its essence. Inversely, the same Quine spoke in connection with functions waiting for their objects as 'semi-twilight entities' in the sense that none of them possess any clear identity as long as it is not engaged with any object, that it remains holed by the empty place that qualifies it. If we think, still like Quine, that there is no entity without identity, we must agree that the Fregean functions remain on the edge of an affirmed existence that will only arrive at the furtive moment that they will disappear as such when, once satisfied by an object, they will have produced a meaning and a truth value.

We find a partially identical intuition in the Husserl of *Logical Investigations* when he distinguishes the 'connection of things' and the 'connection of truths', that he holds to be 'indissociable', adding,

> But this obvious indissociability is not an identity. The real existence of things and of connections of things is expressed in truths or the connections of truths that agree with it. But the truth connections differ from the thing connections that are 'really' in them; and we right away find the proof of this in the fact that these truths applying to truths do not coincide with the truths applying to things posed in these truths.[24]

It is finally, *last but not least*, the Lacanian symbolic which, as treasury of signifiers, prescribes that these arrangements should be conceived of in a certain independence from the real and/or imaginary order that they are supposed to 'represent' (for the function of representation, however decisive it may be in the economy of the subject, is not foundational of the symbolic order as Lacan proposes it).

In all these cases (and others, sometimes quite differently inspired – e.g. Popper and his 'third world'), there is stated an autonomy of knowledge with respect to a referent at which it does not cease to aim to produce sense and meaning. This level of knowledge conceived 'apart' from its possible denotations possesses its exigencies, its local rules of validation, and, above all, a specific property that no one ever had an idea of before someone succeeded in isolating it as such: incompleteness.

The effects of internal limitation

The choice of Lacan's style of maximal resituates us right away in these complex (but at the same time vivifying) coordinates where the universals (the concepts) go their way, respond to one another, overlap one another, intersect one another, clash with one another and contradict one another. In this conceptual network, tensions are organised which demand to be read, without there being any need to precipitate oneself to offer them the shelter of particular existences. When a reader animates this web in however small a way, something happens, in effect, very like the putting to work of a tongue: a sort of general credit is right away opened according to denotation. It is not necessary to brandish in the second a referent to assure a sense. One speaks, and that is valid even before it is proved that one is indeed talking about *something*. Walter Benjamin weighed his words in stating this fact:

> The word must communicate *something* (outside of itself). This is really the original sin of the linguistic spirit. Insofar as it communicates to the outside, the word is in a way the parody by the explicitly mediate verb, of the explicitly immediate verb.[25]

That the concept, like the word, can act as a mediation in speaking about something contributes here the qualifier of parodical with regard to its pure declaring, its explicit and jaculatory immediacy. The poet in Benjamin forces the trait here, but – yes, it is quite true – there can be something grotesque in this mediate function of the verb, in its wish to be forgotten and to only operate intermediaries to highlight something other than itself. This apparent modesty, this obligingness that no one can do without, extinguishes a glimmer which depends on the simple manifestation of the sign, before any relating to anything whatsoever, which Charles Sanders Peirce named for his part the *firstness* of the sign, that he described in this way:

> The idea of the absolutely First must be entirely separated from all conception of or reference to anything else; for what involves a second is itself a second to that second. The First must therefore be present and immediate, so as not to be second to a representation. It must be fresh and new, for if old it is second to its former state. It must be initiative, original, spontaneous, and free; otherwise it is second to a determining cause. It is also something vivid and conscious; so only it avoids being the object of some sensation. It precedes all synthesis and all differentiation; it has no unity and no parts. It cannot be articulately thought; assert it, and it has already lost its characteristic innocence; for assertion always implies a denial of something else. Stop to think of it, and it has flown! . . . That is first: present, immediate, fresh, new, initiative, original, spontaneous, free, vivid, conscious, and evanescent. Only, remember that every description of it must be false to it.[26]

We are dealing here with a limit, which does not suffer any realisation since it claims to aim at something that would stay outside any representation. Peirce needs all his verve to give it existence, needs to make the tongue vibrate to sustain its signifying face without binding it too quickly to a reference that would fully constitute it as a sign. There is scarcely no other recourse to reach such an objective than to pile on meanings, to heap them up until one is out of breath, to ruin any bi-univocal sign/referent relation, and, in this way, to let there be understood a function of the tongue most often deafened by the representative convoy.

Benjamin, to end up with the quotation that we have read, used another stratagem to produce, for his part also, a pure manifestation free of any reference to a goal but determined: anger.

> An unmediated function of violence . . . is already revealed in the experience of daily life. With man, anger, for example, provokes in him the most visible explosions of a violence which is not linked as a means to an end already fixed. It is not a means but a manifestation.[27]

This varied obsession of the immediacy of the signifying manifestation is one of the rare indications that can be advanced to judge the exception as quality and not as (negligible or hyperbolic) quantity. In these attempts (Peirce, Benjamin), we, in effect, witness a sort of determined exhaustion of the concept which does what it can to designate what escapes from its orbit, what refuses designation: this existence of an object which is not one of a sign which is not one, but such that, without it, without that, it's good-bye to signs and objects! Farewell to the endless mediations of meaning and the meanderings of the representative process.

We will have been careful not to forget here that this is precisely the function devolved by Lacan onto his **o**-object whose initial statement of work carried the mention, via the Kantian *nihil negativum*, of not falling under any concept. Why such a requirement, if not to set aside whatever can be deferred in any referential use of a sign, of a concept? This secondarity, denounced by Peirce in his research of a firstness which would be such, Lacan also, in his way, sets it aside with his object, just as Benjamin in his entanglements with the forms of violence in law; all three attempt to give a status in the order of knowledge to a *manifestation without any mediation*, a manifestation present at the heart of the representative process without the latter ever in capacity to catch it, while it constantly claims to do so with each and every thing.

Here comes what is most delicate. None of these three authors wants to take up again the romantic complaint about the *outer* limits of the world of representation, about the fact that the concept seems to allow to escape the most precious part of what it claims to circumscribe, that the portrait always misses its model, ignores life in its mysterious incarnations, and so on. Of course, from here and there, one will find some accent of this so orphic, so poetic (see Bonnefoy discussed earlier) complaint, but it is not constitutive of their position. It is much more a matter of correctly localising what constitutes an exception to the regime of representation, otherwise eminently useful, but which of itself proves to be incapable of recognising the inner limitations of the symbolic systems that it puts to work to constitute knowledge. Perhaps the word *limitation*, banal in logic, is deceptive here in what it suggests in terms of handicap, of restriction of the field of action, while it only serves to state the very consistency which allows this knowledge to operate *ad libitum* in the field of representation.

The exception that these formulae quite clearly separate out thanks to the maximal particular, with its particular affirmative ($\exists x.\overline{\Phi x}$) which visibly goes against the universal of the same name, is therefore not to be considered numerically but plastically, insofar as it manifests this existence which gives form to traits. While in the minimal particular affirmative ($\exists \mathbf{x}.\Phi \mathbf{x}$), these traits ($\Phi \mathbf{x}$) take the ascendancy over the existence of this form by blending in the resemblance with the model or the specific identity stated at the level of the universal ($\forall \mathbf{x}.\Phi \mathbf{x}$), in the maximal particular affirmative ($\exists x.\overline{\Phi x}$), the affirmation of existence comes into the foreground, without having to attach itself to the presence of universalised traits. But at the same time, this exception is also the poorest imaginable: we can say nothing about it, we are only allowed to affirm it – and even then, we have seen that Peirce, in his dishevelled rigour, rhetorically refused it.

The extreme point reached here also bears in logic the appellation of the 'elimination of singulars'. No settling of accounts or genocide in perspective: it is only a matter of getting rid of the problems linked to the question of the reference of singular nouns (*noms*). If I affirm 'Socrates was Plato's master', I am confusing in the name 'Socrates' a conviction about his existence and the fact that he was Plato's master. Now a whole movement of modern symbolic logic has tended to make this duality explode and to distinguish the brute fact of existence and the predicate that one wishes to attribute to it. In so doing people try to separate out from logical calculus the ontological *a prioris* that do not belong to it and graft on to it considerations that reduce its possible developments (this movement begins with Frege and his *Begriffschrift*, and once started, nothing stops it). It was therefore agreed to say rather: there exists an x such that x is Socrates and such that this x was Plato's master:

$$\exists x.\ (x = \text{Socrates});\ (x = \text{Plato's master})$$

In this way, the space of the calculus is separated out by isolating, through writing, its existential hypotheses, as if by a sort of common factorising. This is moreover the work of the maximal particular affirmative promoted by Lacan ($\exists x.\overline{\Phi x}$): it distinguishes the existant and the calculation that besides it deploys, in the operation of traits and functions, from their negations, conjunctions and other implications. The existant finds itself posed separately, ex-tracted (*ex-trait*) from the symbolic determinations that it supports, which eventually determines it on its journey but with which it is not confused.[28] This x deserves to be called 'subject', even if this *hypokeimenon* suitable for supporting predicates is no longer here inflated by some substance or other. How respect its consistency once one claims to value it?

The forced aspect of the clinical vignette comes from the fact that it fails here almost in principle: if the *x* is only so convoked under the heading of the relevance of the traits that it displays, it will never be anything more than the shadow cast by the concepts whose colours it defends (willingly or unwillingly). How then approach it in order to allow it its place, since there is no question of plunging into the negative theologies of the subject and of praising its merits along the style of 'Thou wilt always escape us'? The maximal particular here opens up a track, which might well convey a different clinic.

On the Freudian case and its rapport to the universal

Freud happens to have left to his posterity a text in which, from the title, he inscribes he places himself in the frame of our maximal particular since he takes up the challenge of 'a case of paranoia that contradicts the theory'.[29] How does he get out of this opposition to a conceptual construction with pretensions to universality that he himself had taken the trouble to produce?

Four years after the writing of the Schreber case, he is, in effect, in possession of his thesis on paranoia, already sketched out at the time of his rupture with Fliess: the paranoiac 'struggles against the reinforcement of his homosexual tendencies', in such a way that, because of a certain number of annexed considerations and reasonings, the persecutor must be of the same sex as the persecuted. Now the female patient – that a lawyer friend of Freud has brought him – presents an undeniable delusion where the persecutor is, in just as obvious a way, a man. 'We did not maintain, it is true', Freud then writes, '*as universal and without exception* valid the thesis that paranoia is determined by homosexuality; but this was because our observations were not sufficiently numerous'.[30] Here is something that sounds like an appeal to induction: his study of the Schreber case had indeed met with a certain consensus from those around him, but this does not seem to have sufficed here for Freud-the-scientist, with his position of only endorsing his hypotheses if they have been confirmed by numerous experiments. Moreover, he immediately drives his point home, not without entering into the general problematic of cases:

> The thesis was one of those which in view of certain considerations become important only when universal application can be claimed for them in psychiatric literature there are certainly no lack of cases in which the patient imagines himself persecuted by a person of the opposite sex. It is one thing however to read of such cases and quite a different thing to come into personal contact with one of them.[31]

The authority of the thing seen takes precedence here over the 'literature', as it is *de rigueur* in good clinical practice where the sign is first apprehended in its context. Freud hastens therefore to summon the young woman for a second time, the lawyer being from now on outside the affair. She, for her part, is not asking for anything, shows herself right away distrustful, and afterwards does not come back. She nevertheless accepts this second conversation that Freud forces on her, courteously but firmly it seems.[32] 'The additional details she supplied', Freud immediately writes, 'resolved all doubts and difficulties'. In effect, there then appears behind the masculine character who is in the position of official persecutor another character, an elderly lady (with white hair, like her mother).

The patient considers that she has reasons to suppose that this woman has received from the man some confidences concerning the timid beginnings of a sexual life between the two of them. With these new data in his possession, Freud rediscovers right away his Oedipal markers:

> It is easy to see that the white-haired elderly superior was a substitute for her mother, that in spite of his youth her lover has been put in the place of her father, and that it was the strength of her mother complex which had driven the patient to suspect a love-relationship between these ill-matched partners, however unlikely such a relation might be.

Because of this, the contradiction with psychoanalytic theory vanishes, evaporates (*verflüchtigt*), and the thesis about the homosexual roots of paranoia emerge quite cheerfully: the real persecutor is the elderly woman, therefore of the same sex as the patient! There nevertheless remains to be explained the displacement which made a change in the delusion from the old woman to the young man. Here, Freud's article suddenly becomes more complicated and more interesting. Up to now, Sherlock Holmes has won out: the clinician has not let himself be undone and was able to rediscover under the deceptive tinsel of appearances, the truth of the profound connections which have produced the situation under observation. Freud is by this very fact all the more at home in that he has rediscovered not simply his Oedipal model but also, and above all, his fundamental schema of intervention, which had acquired paradigmatic value ever since the *Interpretation of Dreams*: take a text, consider it as the manifest face of another latent text, and once this latter has been exhumed (reconstructed?), explain the passage from the latent to the manifest, and you will see how the censor has intervened to allow it to get through without repression being lifted.

Abandoning psychosis for a moment, Freud regains the field of the neurosis to remark that some neurasthenics, because of their unconscious liaison with an object of incestuous love, cannot approach an unknown woman and must content themselves, in this respect, with what their phantasmatic life offers them. But on that terrain – and here is the add-on that throws light on the case of paranoia – these same neurasthenics can very well succeed in substituting an unknown woman for the mother or for the sister. They therefore succeed on the plane of reverie what remains forbidden to them in acts, and in this way, they can convince themselves that they are in love with women outside the family circle. Scarcely has he posed this consideration than Freud enlarges the debate: Does the symptom always make the neurotic conflict disappear? Yes, but in fact no:

> Indeed we can hardly draw any conceptual distinction between these two classes of phenomena. We are too apt to think that the conflict underlying a neurosis is brought to an end when the symptom has been formed. In reality the struggle can go on in many ways after this. Fresh instinctual components arise on both sides, and these prolong it. The symptom itself becomes an object of this struggle; certain trends anxious to preserve it conflict with others which strive to remove it and to re-establish the *status quo ante*.[33]

People of bad will who might try to catch Freud out on the fact that a theoretical forcing would be here, have their work cut out: thanks to a double somersault, he rediscovers his hypotheses in such a way that being in possession of such a complex theory and of such a pragmatic clinical attitude, one feels that in the end he will always be right and will manage to get out of any eventual contradictions. But it is of little interest to us to criticise him in this way for what is important is precisely the rebound which forces him to this add-on which, going far beyond the contradictory case, puts in question the first affirmation according to which the symptom puts an end to the neurotic conflict that gave birth to it.

'There are', writes Freud, 'many similar processes occurring outside paranoia which have not yet been looked at from this point of view'.[34] It is therefore decisive that the article does not stop on the rediscoveries of the Oedipus complex and of the persecutor of the same sex but that the interpretative paradigm coming from the work on the dream relegates the latent content (constructed in grand part by theoretical convictions) to a role that is certainly necessary but nevertheless subalternate. When Freud rediscovers his theoretical markers in this case, he is more or less as far advanced as when in the writing of the *Interpretation of Dreams*, he notices that he is dealing with one of his numerous dreams inspired, at that time, by his wish to be named as extraordinary professor. He does not despise them; he knows only that the latent content is not the alpha and the omega of his work: nothing but a stage in the process of deciphering which must account for the passage from *this* latent to *this* manifest.

His convictions on the homosexual foundations of paranoia (and not the paranoiac foundations of homosexuality!) are not of the order of hypotheses which could be invalidated by cases, despite the presentation that he gives of them. This posture of the honest scientific experimenter, that Freud quite often affects, masks the semiotic and epistemological situations in operation. As regards the first, the presence of signifieds (in a latent position) are not enough for the signifying distribution observed (in a manifest posture): that the persecutor should be, in the end, of the same sex as the persecuted does not constitute a point of arrest from which the Freudian clinician might have peace of mind since he still has to account for the displacement which allows there to be adjusted what is clinically observed and the theory that predicts it.

As regards the epistemological situation, it is fairly clear: Freud, with all due respect, is never in the situation of a Bachelard, or a Popper, in which a polemical fact can, just by itself, bring down a theory by obstinately resisting all the explanations that it proposes for it. He is, on the contrary (the case here studied in this respect 'is a vignette'), in an epistemological situation known under the name of the 'Duhem–Quine thesis' in which a single fact duly tested cannot invalidate the totality of theoretical statements that have participated in its production. Duhem had stated this thesis from the beginning of the 20th century relatively to physical theories, and Quine took it up again in the middle of the same century to give it its logical foundation.[35] The attachment of analysts to their theories being at least as lively as that of scientists to theirs, it is ruled out that we should see, on the level of cases, crucial combats that would allow one theory to be invalidated in favour of another. One can at the very most note the different cravings of each theory for particular types of case: phenomenological psychiatry has written its most beautiful pages on melancholy and states of mania, Freudian psychoanalysis excels on hysteria, behavioural therapies hold fast to the phobias, Winnicottians have an affection for the supposed borderlines, and so on. Each seems to lose a bit of its relevance by enlarging too much its field of action as regards cases, obliged as it then is to become more complex, sometimes to excess; none of them cover a hypothetical 'field of psychopathology', delimited for its part by norms that escape as much from each one as from the unthinkable 'alls'. We should take this point as a given and seek starting from there the status that can be granted to our $\exists x.\overline{\Phi x}$.

Passing through Crete

By reading only the left-hand side of the logical square of the maximal particular, $\exists x.\overline{\Phi x}$ encounters the paradox of Epimenides the Cretan, stating the universal affirmative according to which 'all Cretans are liars': $\forall \boldsymbol{x}.\boldsymbol{\Phi x}$. This universal, which supports a supposedly truthful theoretical statement about a generic plural – the Cretans – is stated by some x who does not claim for all that to escape, either from the totality to which he belongs or from the law that he states as a truth and according to which he himself would be a liar. Now, in so doing, he really does intend to tell the truth in this respect and positions himself therefore as this x who, while stating a universal, contradicts it by this very stating $\exists x.\overline{\Phi x}$.

In order to read this paradox, to make it resonate beyond the refrain to which it is often limited by being satisfied to mention it, we must, first of all, become sensitive to the redoubling of the quality in operation here: logical formulae, whatever they may be, all claim to be either true or false according to whether the predicate is or is not in the subject (at least in classical logic, but we are deliberately keeping to this frame), and this is what we will agree to call their 'value'. But here we have the proposition of Epimenides, not content to have, like all its consœurs, a truth-value, also intending to make of the truth the predicate of the subject that it requires. Are we truthful when we tell the truth? The least domestic quarrel would be enough to know that this is not so: by telling the truth, one can do a lot of other things, as

Nietzsche had already become noticed (take power, corner one's interlocutor, try to be smart, satisfy the gods, etc.). What then is Epimenides doing when he affirms a mode of relationship of Cretans (therefore of himself) to the truth in an assertion which has also, on its own account, something to do with the truth? Let us imagine that he had said instead 'all Cretans are big' and that the testimonies agreed in letting us know that he was rather small for his time and his milieu: no problem – all Cretans are big (Epimenides says so, and we have our own reasons to trust him), except him. He constitutes an exception in the most banal sense of the term, and it's all settled: take all those who possess the predicate, and add all those who do not possess it (but are picked out under this heading)[36] and you have an all, *tous* (all) perfectly sound.

With the truth in the position of predicate *and* in the position of value, a chiasm is produced which gives the statement all its charm in that it awaits our verdict, if at least we set aside a reading that would only take account of the simple predicate (as earlier with size), and we treat the matter numerically by considering that all Cretans are liars except Epimenides – but then we envisage the fact of telling the truth uniquely as a psychological property, that one can possess or not, the Cretans yes, Epimenides no. If, on the contrary, one considers together the truth as value of the proposition and the truth as predicate of the subject, then we fall feet first into the paradox formally presented by the structure of Russell's paradox: if Epimenides tells the truth, there is at least one Cretan excluded from the universal in which they are collected, therefore the universal proposition is false and Epimenides is telling a falsehood (he is lying) when he states it; if he is lying, he rejoins the lying Cretans; therefore, all are so, which makes the statement of the universal proposition true, and therefore he is telling the truth . . . when he is lying.[37] If he is right, he is wrong; if he is wrong, he is right. This turnstile offers no exit.

The 'sets that do not belong to themselves', dear to Russell and fatal for Frege, dance the same jig: if they belong to themselves, they do not belong to themselves, and if they do not belong to themselves, they belong to themselves. All that because *belonging* is a noun to designate the link between the set and its elements, just as truth designates the nature of the link between the subject and its predicate (for the proposition in classical logic) or between the function and its object (in Fregean logic). However little such properties are, as it were, folded back on themselves to participate in their own gestation there follows a local disturbance, which nevertheless threatens the whole of the edifice.

In the light of the preceding, what are we to think of $\exists x.\overline{\Phi x}$ as a 'hopeless requirement' ('*requisit désespéré*') having in view an 'at least one' that is not a slave to the phallic function, not submitted to castration (equivalent formulae for Lacan)? For all are so! It is useless therefore to arm oneself with an *Urvater*, an originating father, after having set aside without appeal an 'all women' since, being implied in one another, these two statements are logically equivalent. The exception no longer designates here any element that would be extracted from the set for which the universal is valid any more than Epimenides does not cease to be a Cretan by decreeing that they are all liars.

An exception that would not be a 'case'

Let us now recapitulate the characteristics encountered around this exception cornered in the formulae of sexuation in the position of the particular maximal affirmative. It is not singular or even in a minority with respect to the universal affirmative that it wrong-foots. It is produced only as a contradiction of the universal negative which, for its part, would be an affirmation of the 'nothing' that Lacan has pursued from the beginning, this nothing which is neither that of Hegel nor that of Freud, the very absence of subject about which one can predicate. It is therefore, first off, an affirmation of what exists with respect to the function (of the predicate), without for all that satisfying it (possessing it). So then, far from being based on a supposed rarity, the exception veers towards the common regime and every speaking being, linked by this fact to the phallic function, becomes a sort of sexual Epimenides, lending its voice to the establishment of this all (*tous*) to which it belongs, but whose consistency it ruins by its very declaration, neither more nor less than any living being in the process of stating 'all men are mortal' not without arranging for himself *in petto* room for an exception – the one that religions trade on.

Here let us thank Abelard for having offered us early on the refuge of his *status*, for having suggested to us the idea according to which between . . . let us say things, for want of anything better, and the sonorous (or scriptural) nature of words, there exists, there is, we suppose, entities which allow individuals to be collectivised, without nevertheless their enjoying any ontological weight whatsoever. It is really what we need to appreciate the proper weight of $\forall x.\Phi x$, *once one asks oneself who is saying it, who is performing it.*

For the question posed by the exception that Lacan is circling comes back to the mysteries of belonging (from which Russell's paradox is generated): we have seen that, to use the quantifier ∀ ('for any'), it was necessary to have a set peopled by elements that belong to the aforesaid set. On this condition, it was permitted to take any one of them with these tweezers of the ∀ ('for any'). But if I affirm the existence of (at least) one which does not satisfy the function ($\exists x.\overline{\Phi x}$), which in this way is excepted from the all of the universal, does it cease belonging to this all? Yes and no (Freud would say)!

Logic cannot be constructed on such ambiguity and settles the question: in the logical square of the maximal, either the universals are true or the particulars are true, but it is ruled out that a universal and a particular should be true at the same time because they are linked by a contradiction. With Lacan, as with Epimenides, there is on the contrary preserved an essential ambiguity in the measure that, because of the function (or of the predicate) at stake, the truth of the particular statement does not annihilate the truth of the universal statement, since, on the contrary, it establishes it by the very fact of objecting to it (*dixit* Lacan, cf. the previous discussion) by providing it with the existent that states it, that lends its voice to the declaration of this universal from which nonetheless it is lacking. But with his logical square, Lacan, all the same, tells us more about it than the Cretan who, for his part, does not have a good word to say for the female Cretans.

He, in effect, gives himself a 'woman' side where any exception finds itself denied ($\overline{\exists x}.\overline{\Phi x}$), where therefore the way of writing proposed for the universal negative affirms that, in this *deixis*, there does not exist any x that does not satisfy the function at the very time that the elements which satisfy it present only at the level of the particular negative do not constitute a set. To recall the formula proposed as a conclusion to the preceding chapter: *inasmuch as an all is stated* ($\forall x.\Phi x$), *it is founded on the existence of exceptions* ($\exists x.\overline{\Phi x}$), *and inasmuch as there is no exception* ($\overline{\exists x}.\overline{\Phi x}$), *what exists is not collectivised in any all* ($\overline{\forall x}.\Phi x$). In both cases, the all takes a hit. The universality of the concept, which finds its basis in that very all, is nonetheless manhandled by it (even though differently) on the left and on the right, and we realise then that the not-all goes beyond its quality of quantifier in giving the reason for the set of formulae.

Lacan's merit comes from the fact of letting himself be guided by the exigencies of this particular by forcing himself to write each of his four positions in a way that allows there to be read there from the start the attack directed against an 'all' that would possess any ontological weight whatsoever. This leads consequently on the epistemic plane, to the status that it is appropriate to grant to the concept in this teaching of his: the precision that the concept requires (and of which it is often the object) says nothing about the reality of its possible denotations. Between the concept and the individuals that might fall within its orbit (something which obviously is not denied, the minimal particular continues to work just as well), there will remain active this **o**-object which, for its part, depends entirely on the maximal particular does not fall under any concept and maintains itself as existence without essence, an existence decisive in the subjective process.

There is another consequence that I deliberately left to one side since attacking these formulae, for fear that the imaginary weight of the terms utilised – man/woman – would charge the ways of writing with unwarranted values in order to pretend to find them afterwards. Now that we have glimpsed the solidarity of the left and the right sides in this logical square that we continue to call the 'formulae of sexuation', in what way does one deserve to be called 'man' and the other 'woman'?

Did you say 'rapport'?

In the Christian tradition, the sexual rapport is indeed always such since every sexual act possesses a value. Either there are fecundation and birth, and the child is the value which results from this relationship, or there is a sexual act without reproduction, but in the sacrament of marriage (and according to the prescribed rules), and this becomes a duty, 'conjugal duty'. For all the rest, if there is a sexual act, whatever it may be, it is sinful. Therefore, every case of a relation held to be sexual is entitled to the name 'rapport' in the sense that interests Lacan, the mathematical sense, when one writes: a/b = c. If two terms enter into relation in such a way that they produce a unique value, then there is a 'rapport'. How to write that such is not the case when, mindful of the Freudian saying which breaks all pre-established harmony between the drive and its object, we refuse to consider any 'reproductive instinct' whatsoever that would take as given a 'nature' of the rapport between the sexes, on a basis that would henceforth see itself as hormonal, or genetic, or anything else whatsoever, preferably of a really scientific style?

Therefore, it comes down to the 'man' to declare the universal affirmative but, moreover, in doing this, to withdraw himself from it, in this wheeling around that we have just seen. To follow Lacan, man supports the universal of the same name by reason of his own defection at this level. He produces the essence of his being while objecting right away by his existence. The 'anything but that', a scream if there ever was one of this same man faced with castration, here takes on the form of an 'anyone, but not me' which proves to be the condition *sine qua non* for all this calibre to be declared. This donation of a universal is brought about by the withdrawal of its particular, which is excluded from the all the better to pose it in its classificatory virtuality. There is here a turning movement lacking which we exhaust ourselves enumerating the contradictions present in the formulae: every 'one' that is excepted from the all the better to perform it (*le performer*) deserves to be qualified as 'man', whatever may be the sex that nature may have attributed to that human being.

In whose name, in these conditions, name 'woman' the position according to which the elements which satisfy do not form any all, without generating the least exception? What imaginary lends itself to this symbolic distribution? For the contradiction is striking: If there is no exception, how can those present not form an all? The response forces itself on us: that each one is not as one as all that, that their gathering together does not seem right, that each existence affirmed in this way (by the particular negative, the 'not-all' ($\overline{\forall x}$) having the value of 'there exists' ($\exists x$) which would display its restrictive value) is either in excess or in default with respect to unity – a Lacanian theme if there was ever one since in this teaching unity emerges, either from a specular (unian, *unienne*) or from the symbolic (unary, *unaire*) value. This indeed is why no value, neither symbolic nor imaginary, will be right to qualify an element in the measure that none will here be identical to itself (otherwise this identity would be enough to integrate into the 'all' of a set).

With all due respect to feminists who may feel themselves attacked by such a distribution of tasks, and far from being a loss as compared to the symbolic unity put on the side of 'man', this dissonance on the right finishes the work engaged on the left by inscribing in the order of sexual determination this **o**-object which we have seen leads to the statement 'there is no sexual *rapport*' precisely because with it 'there was no rapport', not even this very elementary one of possessing this stump of unity that would have made it suitable for the stamp of concept, and by that of entering into relation, of 'making a rapport'.

In this way the left/right, man/woman, ways of writing have the ambition of expressing the fact of non-rapport by placing side by side an x whose functioning allows us to think an essence ($\forall x$) and an existence ($\exists x$), and an x whose functioning does not authorise any essence but is entirely based on an existence which remains resistant to any unity whatsoever. At this price, one can always write man/woman or the reverse, this will give us nothing, no value to mark the existence of a rapport. To make a rapport, at the level of essences one is lacking, and each of the existences classified to the left or to the right is said to be incommensurable to the other. The numerical and set metaphor which served to arrange the man/woman deixis maintains us in the ir-rational, the non-rapport, no common term coming to subsume the putting into relation – for Lacan holds firmly then to his definition of the rapport inasmuch as it produces a tertiary term. Neither the child nor the drive and still less the phantasy plays this role, and therefore, the sexual encounter – which is, of course, undeniable – connects two beings which neither make one nor make three. The phallus, the all-purpose object of Freudian dialectic, is henceforth disqualified as a tertiary element;[38] it disappears into the phallic function which only serves to distinguish and disconnect two functionings irreducible to one another.

Lacan – this is remarkable – was very careful not to write x on the left and y on the right, which he could have done if he had thought for a second that man and woman present themselves as such with such different qualities that they deserve to be written and described separately. On the contrary, it is the same x that is everywhere valid, which everywhere designates the same speakbeing (*parlêtre*) confronted with the enjoyment linked to sex and to language. This little detail draws us still further into the refusal of taking into account an initial duality. Without plunging into a too substantialist conception which would make of this x something ante-sexual, we are thus led to conceive that sexual bipartition results from enunciatory arrangements: the x which is excepted from the all that it poses as the locus of its belonging will be called man and the x which exists without belonging to some all will be called woman. We see that this performative perspective is not in contradiction with Freudian bisexuality for, however different the two positions may be, the one and the other offer themselves to this x with just as much veracity.

To enjoy (*jouir*)

There remains the Φ function, an enigmatic function since, far from being a pure corporeal event, it blends body and spirit much better than the gland – nevertheless pineal – dear to Descartes. Its obscurity grows still more when we learn that the term *enjoyment* (*jouissance*) is quasi-absent in Freud, where the word *Genuss*, that is met with here and there, could be translated in this way, without however ever reaching the concept. To be sure its trace is given in the very Freudian notion of 'beyond of the pleasure principle', but it requires the genius of the French or Spanish tongues to welcome with the greatest naturalness a notion that neither German nor English put into practice so easily. *Jouissance* and *goce* say unambiguously that it is a form of pleasure that is in no way pleasure in the Freudian sense, this more or less brutal lowering of tensions which almost led Freud to the 'Nirvana principle' but, on the contrary, a form of the intensification of certain tensions, those whose anticipative liberation will be the source of pleasure. While waiting for this deliverance, *jouir* raises the stakes, along paths that turn to account the body and its different erogenous zones as well as the symbolic machinery that allow there to be forged desiring postures, to convoke the phantasies considered by Lacan, at a certain epoch of his teaching, as 'that by which desire condescends to pleasure'.

But enjoying (*le jouir*) does not develop only these orgiastic perspectives. We also suppose it to be at the heart of the symptom, in what strengthens repetition, confers on it this absurd force that wants to obstinately go over again the signifying traces that often ageless desires once opened up. In both cases, however, the same soldering is at work between the determined fragments of the symbolic installation and corporeal investments. From then on, there is a great temptation to renew the difference between the sexes by seeking to base it on two disparate modes of enjoying, according to a report whose real foundation we are never sure of, or only results from a certain effect of perspective, like a sort of anamorphosis: penile enjoyment is clearly manifested in its cycle (*érection, éjaculation, détumescence*), vaginal enjoyment being oh-so latent. The first would seem to be as open to observation as sensation; the second, even though it can be noisy, seems, above all, to remain of the order of sensation. And as regards the clitoral, which in our day is refinding some prestige in emerging from its bourgeois, then Freudian, purgatory, however similar it appears to be to the penile, does not possess the obviousness of the phallic cycle. This without prejudice to other erogenous zones, beginning with the rectum, that open up just as many paths to enjoying and enjoyable high points without for all that making a display of their end point, to such an extent that people hasten to uncover in them some 'infinite' or other that would seem to be in confinement here and whose corporeal somersaults quickly pacified would be only a sort of foam, abandoned by the waves of a limitless pleasure on our little private beaches.

Raquel Welch, in her days, when she was a *sex symbol*, did not hesitate to say loud and clear in the feminine media: 'The most important sexual organ for a woman is her brain'. Again, a statement subject to the Duhem-Quine theory, because it is not easy to see what polemical fact, what atrocious experimentation, would invalidate it. But we divine in this remark, authoritative from the point of view of the media, the idea which makes of the rhythm imposed on certain feminine organs nothing other than the musical score waiting for the notes of the melody. It is not a matter of 'thinking' but of 'thoughts' that offer a sense, a direction, to what is happening in the circuits of sensibility . . . and with that seems to designate a *terminus ad quem* for them? A hypothesis! The trouble for anyone who would wish, in effect, to establish here a separate mode of enjoying, comes from the fact that this cerebral quality of a supposed feminine enjoyment scarcely appears absent on the man's side. Masturbation is said there, more than on the other side, to be the 'enjoyment of the idiot', but who will say the degree to which this solitude is acephalic or not? Up to what point could phallic enjoyment – the only one that the formulae take account of[39] – take place without disturbing neuronal networks, without the bringing into play of the language and the images that support it, matrices of phantasmatic postures that free up the approaches to pleasure? No one is satisfied with the mechanics, and we quickly divine the illusion there would be in wanting to classify men and women according to whether orgasm is quicker in the first than in the second. The chronometer will not be of much help in separating out the sexes in function of their style of orgasm.

Might these formulae, with their arid ways of writing, be able to throw some light on this obscure and lightning-like entertainment. Their greatest advantage come from the monotony of this Φx function: whatever it may be, on the one side it is affirmed by the one excepted from it and makes itself the hub of this revolving movement; on the other side, it is experienced by the one that cannot nail down any unity because of it,[40] but it does not change its nature. Might it be a matter of two 'know-hows' with the same function, the difference of organs and of something else or other prescribing two specific, uh, pardon . . . generic . . . no, pardon, opposed modes ways of enjoying? Here is something that would go against our efforts since external qualities would preside over this bipartition! It would be much better to return to our starting hypothesis and to agree that the duality of sexes, with whatever anatomical, psychological, and chromosomatic reality one burdens or decorates it, can only be written by coming up against this fact of language: terms that oppose one another – logical contraries – can moreover be incompatible and therefore separated, only by being bound by a whole chain of relatives and validated by one another. Duality is a concept that itself is irreducibly double, marked by what Lacan distinguished at one time[41] as 'separation' and 'alienation', and then reunited in the figure of a diamond which he makes the operator – fancy that! – of his way of writing the phantasy.

Noting a difference thus comes down to affirming the coexistence of two axes that are themselves contrary, one that states bringing into rapport, the other which poses non-rapport. So that the constant bringing into rapport of every human being with the phallic function can very well go along with the affirmation of the non-rapport between the sexes, of which the formulae give an account. The unfolding of the logical square of the maximal particular comes then to refine the opposition inscribed at the heart of the notion of duality by writing how the sexes are separated and alienated at the same time, in their way of managing the exception, this root of unity. It must be that one of the two should be one by excluding itself from the all, but that the other should also do so is what Lacan rejects. And as regards who makes the one and who makes the other . . .

We cannot conclude without evoking the special poetry that arises from non-rapport itself, for anyone who wants to make of it a concept in its own right, of the hard and exigent kind (we have just seen that it is only the second member of a pair that admits only a clear-cut moiety). In this vein, at the very end of his first seminar at rue d'Ulm, on 24 June 1964, Lacan announced the following:

> The analyst's desire is not a pure desire. It is a desire to obtain absolute difference, a desire which intervenes when, confronted with the primary signifier, the subject is, for the first time, in a position to subject himself to it. There alone may the meaning of a limitless love emerge, because it is outside the limits of the law, where only it may live.[42]

Absolute difference, this time, would be one that magnifies non-rapport, would speak only of it; it would be such that between the two elements that it separates, there would not even be it to make the slightest bond, hence the mythical vein that immediately follows such an impossibility, where we see the subject as on his baptismal-font signifiers. He who will never be anything but represented by a signifier for another (Lacan *dixit*), now lands for an unbelievable first time on the stage that he will never again leave and encounters THE signifier which will mark him with a branding iron. In these lines so often quoted, he who was happy to lampoon the myth of *Totem and Taboo* pays his tribute to the thought of origins, which alone offers him a between-the-two where the first term would be missing. This impossible 'time zero' that anxiety alone renders likely by highlighting it as cause and pushes towards this wild rhetoric (already encountered in Peirce) in which thought, which is only able to produce relations, tries to hand over to the tongue so that it may be able to outline, in its own way and with the means at hand . . . an edge, a true edge, something which is not a frontier, constituted by a lack of neighbourhood which alters its relational capacity, its aptitude for 'entering into rapport'.

In this repetitive attempt to *embody* difference, to isolate non-rapport as an ingredient indispensable for the constitution of the subject, Lacan, in the last years of his teaching, was to come up against on a strange difficulty that he insisted on making his own, and that I propose to visit as what comes to confirm the impossibility of putting one's hand – even if it were topological – on what has the pretension of escaping the concept.

Notes

1 A reminder that when each sex is considered as an essence, it is given a capital.
2 J. Lacan, . . . *ou pire*, 10 May 1972, 15: '[T]his bipartition that is fleeting at every instant, this bipartition between the man and the woman. Everything that is not man . . . is it woman? One might tend to admit it. But since the woman is "notall" why would everything that is not woman be man?'
3 S. Freud, *Three Essays on the Theory of Sexuality*, SE VII 148.
4 For Moreau de Tours and the reproductive instinct, see A. Davidson, *The Emergence of Sexuality: Historical Epistemology and the Formation of Concepts*, Cambridge, MA, Harvard University Press, 2004. For Christian theology, M. Jordan, *The Invention of Sodomy in Christian Theology*, Chicago, The University of Chicago Press, 1997.
5 G. Le Gaufey, *L'incomplétude du symbolique de René Descartes à Jacques Lacan*, Paris, EPEL, 1991, pp. 147–158.
6 The choice of such a statement shows that already in 1962, the reference to Peirce in Lacan was accompanied by a conception of the universal negative equivalent to the universal affirmative. 'There is no man who does not lie' (universal negative) is, in effect, equivalent to 'all men are liars', *omnis homo mendax* (universal affirmative).
7 Taking up again the initiative of Leonhard Euler (1707–1783), who wanted to educate a princess by explaining syllogistic reasoning to her with the help of intersecting and non-intersecting circles, John Venn (1834–1923) generalised them in the form of 'Venn diagrams', which respond to the following definition: 'A schematic representation of sets by closed plane curves without a double point whose interior points are the elements of the set represented, commonly called *patate*'. A. Bouvier, M. George and F. Le Lionnais, *Dictionnaire des mathématiques*, Paris, PUF, 1979, p. 774. In *Le Lasso spéculaire*, Paris, EPEL, 1997, I tried to penetrate a part of the mystery of this *patate*.
8 Blanché, *Structures intellectuelles*, *op. cit.*, p. 59.

9 For example, I do not know of a specific theory of repression in Lacan. His specular ego is not an agency suitable to repress, nor is the 'I' and, still less, the subject. Will it be the signifier itself? Impossible. And therefore, even though he clearly rejects Freud's perception/consciousness ego, he continues to need it to use the notion of repression.

10 Today now that witnesses or historians have produced texts dealing with the same events, one can read some partiality in Freud as narrator. Should we, for all that content with refusing, relent towards him? What relationships between psychoanalysis and history?

11 Example: E. Wagner and R. Gaupp, *Un monstre et son psychiatre*, Paris, Epel, 1996.

12 *Trésor de la langue francaise, TLF*, tome XVI, p. 1145.

13 'In 1963, the French government established by legislation the placing of a vignette on tobacco, designed to contribute 5.5 million francs per year to social security', *Le Monde*, 21 May 1986, p. 21, col.2–3.

14 The poet Jules Laforgue, in his *Imitation de la lune*, written in 1886: 'Absolute, draped with layettes, / At the honeymoon of l'Hymette, / We had far too much the air of vignette!' quoted in the *TLF*, tome XVI, p. 1145. The expression '*faire vignette*' had gone out of fashion, but a certain psychoanalysis is giving it a new lease of life.

15 L. Dethiville, 'Chambre avec vue', in *Les lettres de la SPF* no.14, Paris, SPF-Campagne-Premiere, 2005, pp. 55–67.

16 *Ibid.*, p. 67. Winnicott's sentence presented in this quotation is not a particular reference, except by apparently referring back to *The Fear of Collapse and other Clinical Situations*, mentioned on the preceding page of her article.

17 It would be well to remember here the debates evoked in the first chapter on the question of specific identity and of 'abstractive induction'.

18 W. James, *The Will to Believe* (1896), New York, Dover, 1956, p. 90. (The italics are his.) One might also invoke Dr. Pangloss and Voltaire's *Candide*.

19 Y. Bonnefoy, *Les Tombeaux de Ravenne, in L'Improbable et autres essais,* Paris, Mercure de France, 1993, p. 13.

20 J. Lacan, *Les Psychoses,* Paris, Le Seuil, 1984, p 305. Translation Cormac Gallagher.

21 C. Le Boulengé, 'The formation of analysts: Two orientations', *La cause freudienne. Revue de psychanalyse*, no. 52, November 2002, pp. 4–5.

22 One example among a few is M. Gribinski, 'Furtiva Nox', *Le Démon de l'interprétation, Le fait de l'analyse*, no. 4, mars 1998, pp. 60–65.

23 Is this what made him describe a hyperbolic function as 'exponential function'?

24 E. Husserl, *Recherches logiques I. Prolégomènes à la logique pure* (1900–01), Paris, PUF, 1990, p. 252. Translated by Cormac Gallagher.

25 W. Benjamin, 'On language in general and on human language'. In French: 'Sur le langage humain en général et sur le langage huain', in *Mythe et Violence*, Paris, Denoël, 1971, p. 93.

26 C. S. Peirce, *A Guess at the Riddle of Life*, 1.357.

27 W. Benjamin, 'Critique of Violence', https://english.columbia.edu/files/english/content/Critique_of_Violence.pdf

28 Just as the Freudian quantum of affect, constrained to follow the tribulations of the representation (*Vorstellung*) to which it finds itself soldered (*verlötete*) in its *Vorstellungsrepräsentanz*. The same formal figure.

29 S. Freud, 'A case of paranoia running counter to the psychoanalytic theory of the disease (1915)', SE XIV, pp. 261–272; in German: *Mitteilung eines der Psychoanalytischen Theorie widersprechenden Falles von Paranoïa,* Studienausgabe, vol. 7, Frankfurt, Fischer Verlag, 1973, pp. 207–217.

30 *Ibid.*, p. 265. My italics.

31 '[*A*]*ber es blieb ein anderer Eindruck, von solchen Fallen zu lesen, als einen derselben selbst vor sich zu sehen*'.

32 'I therefore said that I could not form an immediate opinion, and asked the patient to call on me a second time, when she could relate her story at greater length and add any subsidiary details that might have been omitted'. *Ibid.*, p. 266.

33 *Ibid.*, pp. 271–272.

34 *Ibid.*

35 Cf. S. Laugier, *L'anthropologie logique de Quine. L'apprentissage de l'obvie*, Paris, Vrin, 1992, especially the pages devoted to '*La révision impossible*', pp. 199–210.

36 Cf. the earlier discussion regarding the question of the absence of the trait. With the set 'Cretans' being founded, for its part, on a geographical entity other than size or liar, it becomes possible to qualify an individual by the absence of one or other trait, which is not the case of woman in the perspective of the formulae where no set previously collectivises them as such.

37 To lie is presented as a deliberate act, which puts much more psychology into the affair than what classical logic is in a position to take responsibility for. The psychologist, for his part, will not see a great paradox in the fact that someone can tell the truth by lying – or lie in telling the truth, which already is not the same thing.

38 It was, on the contrary, its status at the time of the seminar *Desire and its interpretation*, cf. the previous discussion regarding the quotation at the beginning of Chapter 2.

39 The 'enjoyment of the Other', j(O), makes its appearance late in the seminars, in the course of the Borromean elaboration, as a pendant to phallic enjoyment J(Φ). This goes beyond our reading of the formulae, centred on what it is permitted to do with the simple Φ function.

40 Which also suggests the idea of infinity because what no unity encircles deserves to be considered as a 'multiplicity of multiplicities', an expression that serves sometimes to designate the actual infinity of real numbers. But these references to mathematical realities, however instructive they may be in proposing appellations and images that are not too deceptive, also lead us astray sometimes by taking as a guide a knowledge that is too certain, too impressive, which disturbs the operation, all comings and goings, of the metaphor.

41 J. Lacan, *Les Quatre concepts fondamentaux de la psychanalyse*, Paris, Le Seuil, 1973, pp. 190–194.

42 *Ibid.*, p. 248.

4

SCHOLION

A misuse of metaphor

Quite imperceptibly, between 1972 and 1975, Lacan brings about a slippage in the negation regarding sexual rapport, going from 'there is no rapport' to 'there is a non-rapport', from the inexistence of such a rapport to the existence of such a non-rapport. The nuance might appear rhetorical if there were not grafted onto it a change of perspective which takes support on the key instrument in the teaching of these years of the seventies: the Borromean knot.

Towards the end of the seminar *R.S.I.*, Lacan proposes in effect, in this nodular vein, to differentiate 'rapport' and 'non-rapport' by helping himself with two different types of knotting: rapport will be supported by simple concatenation, represented by two closed rings of string, two consistencies which interpenetrate one another, as in the Olympic chain, while non-rapport will, for its part, be supported by the Borromean knotting, by the fact that none of the three consistencies penetrates another one, that none therefore entertains a 'rapport' (in the Olympic sense) with any particular one of the others even though all three are linked. On 15 April 1975, from the beginning of this session, he specifies:

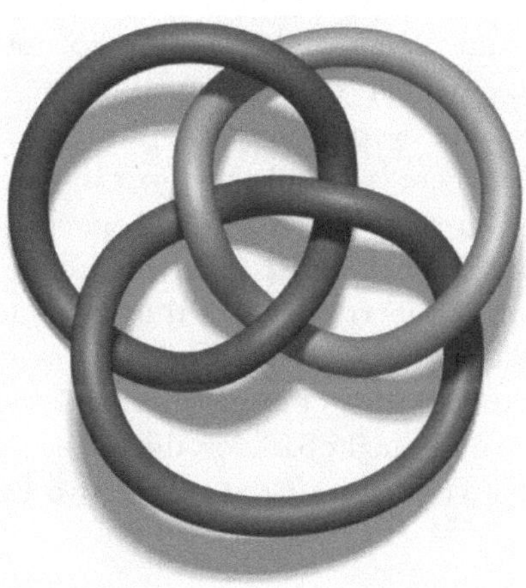

> It is in that [because of the Borromean knotting whose foundational property he has just enunciated: cut one of them and the two others are freed], that the term of sexual non-rapport can be supported insofar as – I can only repeat – it is essentially supported by a non-rapport of couple. Does the enchained knot suffice to represent the rapport of couple?

Non-rapport advances thus in the positivity of a new type of bond, 'this bond that I call the sexual non-rapport', Lacan goes as far as saying the same day,[1] while the term of *rapport* continues to enjoy the positivity that always had, but through the reduced image of direct interpenetration. Henceforth, from fact that in the Borromean knot there is no rapport between two consistencies but only a bond between the three, and *from the fact that the meaning of the word* rapport *had been* (rather silently) *restricted to a couple of elements in which each one is knotted to the other*, this threefold knot comes to designate the non-rapport, to offer it the lodging of a singular representation. To the pure and simple absence of rapport there now succeeds a particular form of the bond which is differentiated from the rapport.

Now this way of doing things formally renews the operation realised at the time of the introduction of unilateral surfaces during the seminar on *Identification*. Lacan, as we saw, then sought to position his o-object outside the narcissistic register (and therefore the specular, the equivalence dates from 1936–1938) to make it exist without for all that endowing it with a mirror image. On what can we base ourselves to make such a thing understood without going as far as identifying it to a mirage or a vampire, the only beings known not to appear in mirrors? With the Moebius strip, the Klein bottle and the cross-cap, Lacan uses surfaces which, of course, possess a mirror image, but this specular image cannot be differentiated from the surface presented in front of the mirror. No matter how you orientate it, the mirror will not invert this orientation and contrary to the right glove which, in the mirror, becomes a left glove, a Moebius strip sporting a straight arrow generates in the plane mirror presented to it a Moebius strip with the same orientation. Lacan – following in this the mathematicians who named such surfaces 'non-enantiomorphic' – then takes the position of considering that they do not have a mirror image, which is only, when all is said and done, an ellipse: they do not have a different one from themselves because of their orientation. But here is something which is enough to indicate that not everything passes through the mirror of specular representation, and thus, there is found the effort to name an object such that it escapes from narcissism since narcissism and specularity go together from the start; specularity has limits because of the existence of unilateral surfaces and their bizarre specular properties, which thus come to plead the cause of a non-narcissistic object.

In the same vein, at the beginning of the seventies and without any great fuss, the word *rapport* sees its domain brought back, on the topological plane, to the simple concatenation of two (or x) interlocking elements (two by two to make a chain or several as in the Olympic knot), and this right away separates out Borromean knotting as the presentification of a type of bond which then deserves to be named 'non-rapport'. Non-specular and non-rapport only assert themselves in this way when their positive terms have been redefined in a sufficiently restrictive way for their negations not to see their sense wavering this way and that and sinking into anything at all or nothing. 'Non-specular' does not designate 'anything that is not specular' but only *anything which possesses an image in the mirror such that one cannot differentiate it from the object itself.* And similarly 'non-rapport' will not designate the pure and simple absence of rapport, but *this type of threefold bond irreducible to two by two liaisons* (apparently, Borromean knotting alone presents this property). We have to wait for the end of the seminar *R.S.I.*, on 13 May 1975, to hear the thing put clearly:

> This in order to make you sense that when I state that there is no sexual rapport, I am giving to the sense of the word 'rapport' the idea of proportion. But everyone knows that Euclid's *more geometricum*, which sufficed for so long to appear the paragon of logic, is quite insufficient and that by entering into the figure of the knot, there is a completely different way of supporting the figure of the non-rapport of the sexes: it is to support them by two circles insofar as they are not knotted. This is what is at stake in what I state about non-rapport. Each of these circles which are constituted, we do not know yet of what, in the rapport of the sexes, each one in its way of going around in circles as sex is not knotted to the other. That is what is meant by my non-rapport.

This clarification is welcome – one can measure its distance compared to the generative instinct (*instinct génésique*) which knotted, without appeal, one sex to the other – but it comes at a price: the object which is worthy of proof must be univocal; one must be able to grasp it without hesitation. Is this indeed the case of the Borromean knot? Do all the presentations of this knot refer to a single and unique object? The question may appear to be idle; Lacan, for his part, shows a singular obstinacy in this connection. Not only does he question himself about his very beginnings in the affair, but he also comes back to it on several occasions, in an always more specific fashion. The 18 March 1975, almost at the end of the seminar *R.S.I.*, noting the discussions going on with Pierre Soury, his principal interlocutor on Borromean questions, he evokes the problem resulting from the fact of distinguishing each of the *R.S.I* consistencies (in colouring them as well as naming them), and this on the basis of his central affirmation on the equivalence of consistencies.

What the Borromean knot with three rings offers him in its physical definition (cut any one of these consistencies, and the two others are freed), is, in effect, three strictly equivalent rings of string which suits him like 'a ring on the finger' since he intends to sustain, over against a previous period of his teaching, that imaginary, symbolic, and real which name each of these rings of string are not ordered in terms of any precedence but should be recognised as having the same value. They must nevertheless be distinguished, because to say they are equivalent does not come down to confusing them or interchanging them. The possibility of colouring them then presents itself: if one endows each consistency with a colour which differentiates it from the two others, will all the presentations that I may give of it be reducible to one and the same knot, or on the contrary am I going to come up against two or several knots irreducible to one another? This 18 March 1975, the question makes its apparition:

> There would be another way – let us not say of recognising these rings, for this would already be to enter into all sorts of implications – let us say differentiating them, which would be to colour them. . . . I had asked the question at one of my preceding seminars, whether these knots – I had taken one, a bit more complicated than the Borromean knot of three, not that they were not three – but I had asked the question of whether this knot was only one, namely, whether the introduction of a differentiation into the knot left the knot, not similar (*pareil*), but always the same. It is effectively always the same, but there is only a single way of demonstrating it: which is to demonstrate that in every case – what is meant by 'case'? – it is reducible to the similar.

Lacan then notes the response that Soury had brought him, and according to which the checking of different ways of flattening out a knot with three coloured consistencies shows (without demonstrating it) that there is only a single coloured knot, that whatever may be the rotations, stretchings, reversals, and other licit operations, every coloured presentation of a knot can be brought back to one and the same agreed presentation. But having scarcely enunciated this point, Lacan launches himself into the account of what he names his 'final adventure', namely the idea that if there is well and truly a single coloured knot, there is a good chance that there will be two of them if, instead of colouring the consistencies, one orientates them:

> In fact I was in effect quite convinced that there is only one coloured knot, but I vacillated – this is what I call my last adventure – about the orientated knot. . . . I did not go so far as to say to myself that there were eight knots, I'm not that stupid! I did not even go so far as to think that there were four of them, but I do not know why I was racking my brains over the fact that there were two of them.

Then he receives the missive from Soury showing that there is only one knot if one orientates each one of the consistencies. Relief on the part of Lacan who, nevertheless takes advantage of it to relaunch the question: to reach his ends, to show that the different presentations of an orientated knot can be reduced to one and the same figure by geometrical operations licit in topological space (no cut, no folding, etc.), Soury has utilised the 'flattening out' of the knot. Far from considering the presentations in their physical reality, in three-dimensional space, Soury sticks them on a plane, writes them with the help of their over/under sequences, and, thanks to that, manages to show that it is always possible to bring these figures back to one and the same drawing in accordance with regulated transformations.

Lacan shows himself very sensitive to this demonstrative detour for, in addition to the question of a threefold knotting, it bears witness to a writing event (*fait d'écriture*). Now the inexistence of the (sexual) rapport then the existence of (the sexual) non-rapport are both, from their start, considered as writing-events. There does not exist between the sexes a rapport, Lacan says, *such that it could be written.* Rediscovering with this flattening-out the dimension of writing, he can then agree that with two consistencies unknotted and nevertheless linked by a third, he holds the right object for representing his non-rapport, when even though one differentiates each one of the consistencies by colour or orientation – and we recall that orientation was decisive in this affair of unilateral surfaces at the beginning of the 1960s.

On 16 December 1975, from the first steps of the seminar *Le Sinthome*, the question remains alive in the sense that Lacan takes careful note of what Michel Thomé and Pierre Soury had managed to show him that if one wishes at the same time to colour and to orient each one of the consistencies, then there are two knots irreducible to one another. 'Which of them is true', Lacan very curiously asks, 'and the true with respect to what is involved in the way the imaginary the symbolic and the real are knotted in what supports the subject'. Three months later, Lacan returns to this point, in a tone which is worth noting:

> So then I must admit to you the following, which is that after assented to what Soury and Thomé had articulated for me, namely that a Borromean chain of three shows itself as supporting two different objects, on condition that the three rings that constitute the aforesaid chain are coloured and orientated, the two being required (what distinguishes the two objects in question in a second phase), after having assented to what they said, but superficially in a way, I found myself in the disagreeable position of having imagined that simply to colour them was enough to distinguish the two objects, this because I had consented quite superficially to what they had brought me the affirmation of.

Lacan's little discovery, in this instance, comes down to seeing that it is not necessary to colour and orientate the three consistencies but that it is enough to colour two of them (the third being so by not being) and to orientate a single one of them. He then produces another depiction of the knot which is almost familiar to him, fabricated by the regulated superposition of two infinite straight lines knotted by a consistency which places the three elements into a Borromean structure:

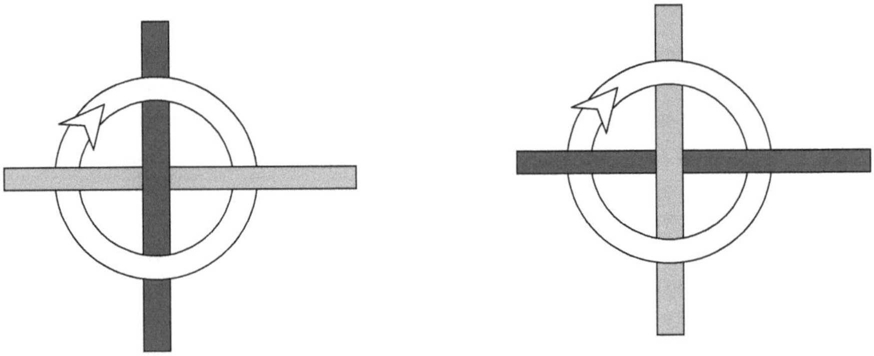

Here therefore are two knots which, with some patience, the reader will be able to convince himself are different, in other words, that no licit operation will allow them to be reduced to one and the same figure or to pass from one to the other. Lacan rather rapidly draws from this some sense-effect:

> The notion of couple, of coloured couple, is there to suggest that in sex, there is nothing more than, I would say, the being of colour. This in itself suggests that there can be *woman the colour of man*, I would say, or *man the colour of woman*. The sexes on this occasion, if we support with the red [white here] ring what is involved in the Symbolic, the sexes on this occasion are opposed as Imaginary and Real, as 'idea' and 'impossible' to take up my terms again.

Already during the preceding session, Lacan had pushed a long way the parallel between nodological accidents and relations between the sexes, basing himself on the following case: let there be a 'faulty' knot, in the form of a trefoil knot, in other words, a Borromean knot whose consistencies have been put in continuity but by making a fault of above/below which makes of the apparent trefoil knot something reducible to a circle. The operations on the knot requiring a minimum of visualisation, the three stages leading to the trefoil knot correctly knotted can be rendered as follows:

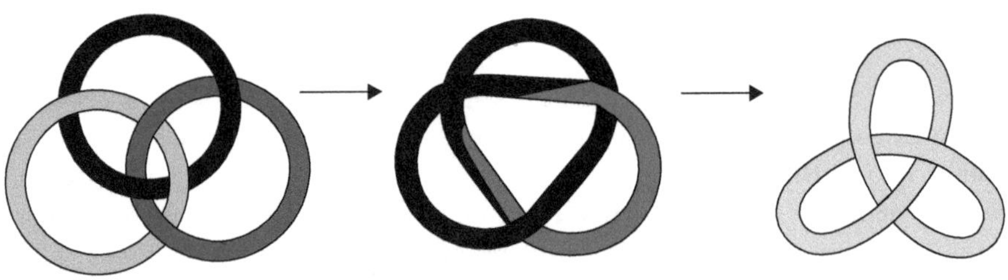

But it may also be that, in the course of this transformation, one commits an error and that one misses out on the completion of the knot, producing with that a false trefoil knot like the one below:

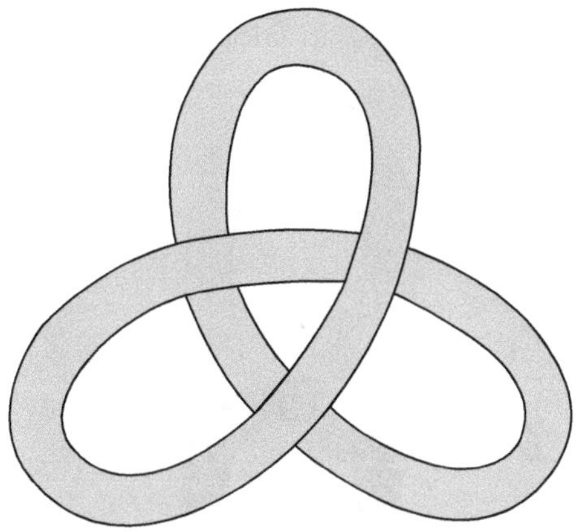

To 'repair' this error and reintroduce a Borromean structure, Lacan introduces another consistency, on the model of the one which he had previously introduced on the level of the classical presentation of the Borromean knot with three consistencies, by the addition of a fourth named '*sinthome*', as is made explicit by the following figure which knots in a Borromean way three circles simply superimposed on one another, since by cutting any one of the four consistencies the three others are freed:

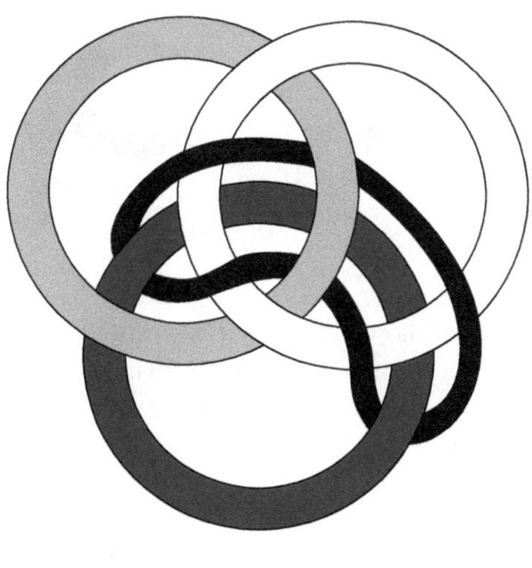

If therefore, armed with this reparation strategy operated with the help of a 'sinthomatic' consistency, one refers anew to the faulty trefoil knot, one sees at the price of a certain effort of reading that the error of above/below is in a way delocalised. It was made at a precise point, but it can be repaired at each one of the three crossing points of the consistencies, with nevertheless consequences that Lacan quite correctly distinguishes. If the repairing takes place at the same place as the error, the knot rediscovers its trefoil structure, as it appears below:

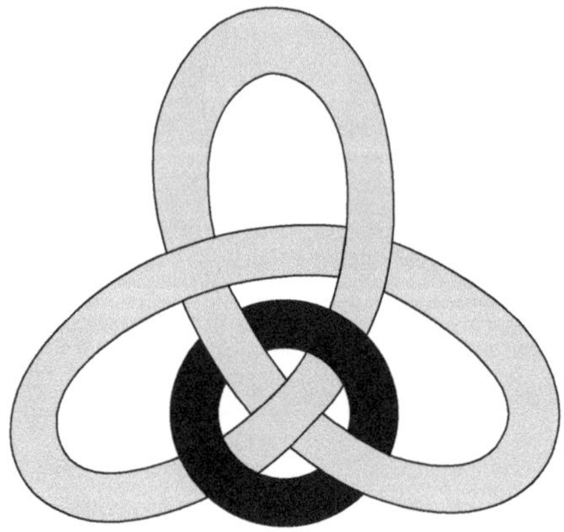

but if it takes place at one or other point of the above–below of the flattening out, the two consistencies which result from it (that of the initial knot and that of the *sinthome*) are interchangeable and therefore equivalent (which was not the case in the repairing at the point of error):

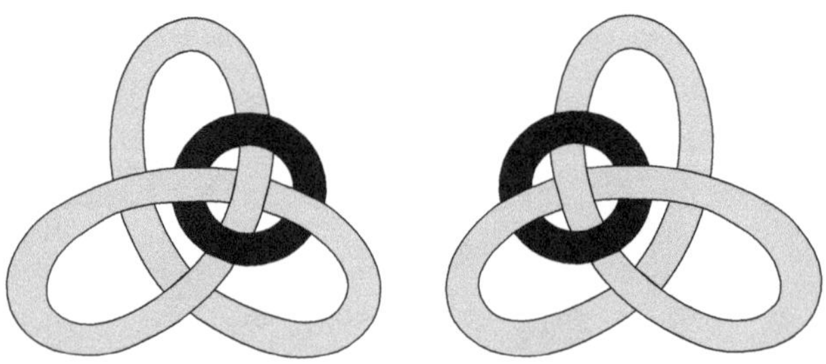

Lacan draws from this the following effect: if the error is repaired at a point other than where it was committed, one will obtain a form of a knot in which the consistencies, from the fact of being strictly interchangeable

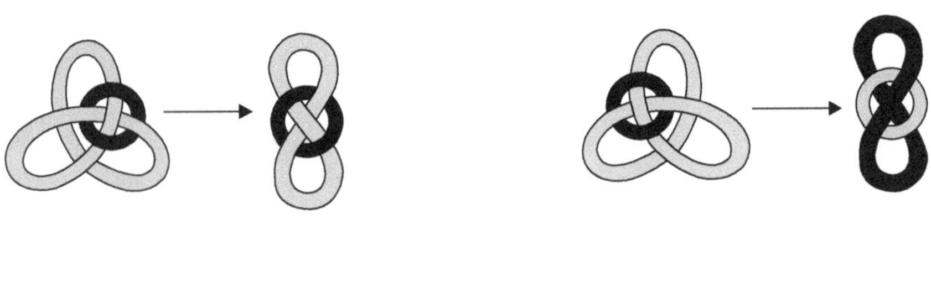

or

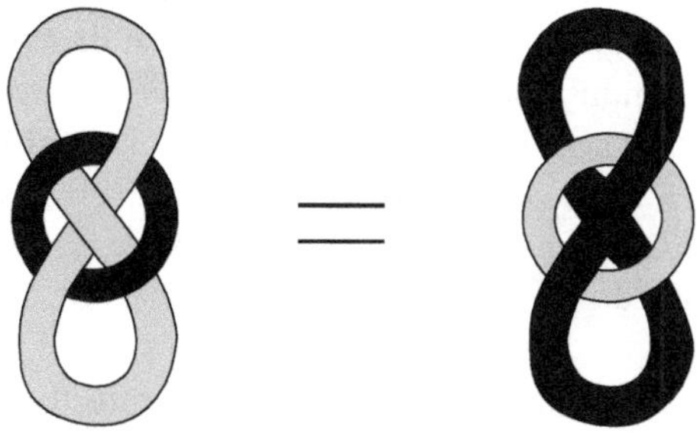

should be considered as equivalent, as opposed to the repairing at the point of error which, for its part constituted the consistencies as non-reducible to one another, not equivalent, and therefore susceptible to entering into 'rapport'. On this point, Lacan shows an imperturbable logic:

> It is in the measure that there is a *sinthome*, that there is no sexual equivalence, namely, that there is rapport; for it is quite certain that if we say that non-rapport depends on equivalence, it is in the measure that there is no equivalence that the rapport is structured. There is therefore at the same time sexual rapport and no rapport, except for the fact that where there is rapport, it is in the measure that there is *sinthome*, namely, where, as I have said, it is by the *sinthome* that the other sex is supported.

One has the impression of having arrived here at the limits of the half-blind procedure to which Lacan is submitting himself, tracking in the properties of the nodological object the asperities from which he is seeking a sense on the side of the sexual non-rapport, allowing a minimal syntax to be given to some key intuitions concerning the sexes, in order to welcome them into a knowledge which respects their difference without hypostasing them.

But at the very time that this duality of the coloured/oriented knot pushes him to these specifications, he holds firmly to the fact that the 'physical' threefold knot, the one in which the three consistencies are strictly equivalent, is unique in its genre:

> To consider now the threefold knot, it is remarkable to note that it does not carry any trace of this difference. But given that it homogenises the Borromean knot, namely, that in it we put the imaginary, the symbolic and the real in continuity, we will not be astonished that we should see that there is only a single one.

This question of unicity does not therefore cease to be at stake in the putting to work of the Borromean knot as 'support' (a word that is very frequent in Lacan in his uses of the knot) of the sexual non-rapport at the same time as it is charged with saying the non-rapport, the absence of direct concatenation, between each of the categories of the imaginary, symbolic, and real. That there is here a metaphor is sure, but Lacan had taken his distance for a long time vis-à-vis metaphor *qua* underpinned by an analogy.[2] There is always room to ask oneself if such a sustained use of this trope is not in his case of a nature to subvert a little bit its sense and its usage. On 20 September 1977, he indicates in his own way the problem with which we find ourselves confronted:

> All that does not tell me how I myself slipped into the Borromean knot to find myself, on some occasions, with a lump in my throat. It must be said that the Borromean knot is what, in thought, constitutes matter. Matter is what one breaks, there also in the sense that this word ordinarily has. What one breaks, is what holds together and is supple on some occasions, like what is called a knot. How did I slip (*glissé*) from the Borromean knot to imagine it composed of tori and, from there, to the thought of turning over each one of these tori, this is what led me to things that constitute a metaphor, a natural metaphor, namely, that that sticks to linguistics inasmuch as there is one. But the metaphor has to be thought of metaphorically. The stuff of metaphor, is what in thought, constitutes matter or, as Descartes says, 'extension', in other words 'body'.

Lacan seeks therefore on the side of the consistency of the knot ('what holds together') properties such that they could 'support' what is involved in the subject, of the imaginary/symbolic/real ternary and in the inexistence of a rapport between the sexes. Since this knot suits locally as a support, how far is it permitted to extend this suitability? On this chapter, Lacan deliberately makes himself a dupe of writing, in a constant metaphorical tension. One can even sometimes believe that psychoanalysis has gone through the trapdoor, lost under the weight of a kind of Borromean erudition, but it surfaces at every moment, questioned henceforth by the knot and its avatars.

On 9 January 1979, at a few cable lengths from the end of this teaching uninterrupted for 27 years, Lacan returns anew – elliptically, as has then become the case in these sessions where his speech has become slow and sparse – on the nature of the relation that he has sustained for almost 10 years between the Borromean knot and his sexual non-rapport. 'There is no sexual *rapport*, this is what I have stated', he recalls from the opening words. 'It is curious', he says a little later, 'that I should have chosen the Borromean knot to make something of it'. Then he engages himself once again in the distinctions between two flattening-outs of the knot that he produces that day and such that they would not be strictly equivalent in their capacity to symbolise imaginary, symbolic, and real. So that while in the two cases the same Borromean knot of three consistencies is at stake, Lacan sets about showing that their flattening-outs, therefore the writings of them that are presented, are not equivalent, that they develop from different plaits.[3] He concludes this ultra-brief session (the stenotype is limited to a page and a half):

> The metaphor of the Borromean knot in its simplest state is incorrect. It is a misuse of metaphor, because in reality there is nothing that supports the imaginary, the symbolic and the real. That there is no sexual rapport, is what is essential in what I state. That there is no sexual rapport because there is an imaginary, a symbolic and a real, is what I did not dare to say. All the same I said it. It is quite obvious that I was wrong, but I allowed myself to slip into it. . . . I allowed myself to slip into it, quite simply. It is vexing, it is even more than annoying. It is all the more annoying in that it is unjustified. This is what appears to me today, and it is at the same time what I am admitting to you. Good!

In a few sentences, the non-rapport – which had the ambition of saying positively the absence of rapport – loses its Borromean support. There is no 'thing' to support such a . . . concept? Inasmuch as one tries to write with the help of the Borromean knot, the unicity of this knot refuses itself, ruining the equivalence sought between a sexual order that one wants to rebel against binarity, and this emblematic Borromean writing of an irreducible triplicity, that cannot be decomposed into dualities. There no longer remains anything but the fragility of a statement – 'there is no sexual *rapport*, this is what I stated. . . . That there is no sexual *rapport*, is the essential of what I state' – to sustain a singular hiatus between the sexes. That same day, in the few sentences that this session involves, Lacan comes to evoke the possibility of a third sex, that he does not comment on any further, contenting himself to add, 'Why is it that there are two of them, moreover, is hard to explain'.

The end of a metaphorical epic, which sometimes took on an allegorical allure, stretched between two orders of knowledge that Lacan forces to advance in such a way that the steps of the one are moulded on the steps of the other. In this journey, the knot has not only exercised our minds with an unusual triplicity (since thinking comes down to concatenating two ideas, advance at the little trot of binarity), but it suggests, moreover, escapees, questions obvious things in another knowledge, the psychoanalytic one, which has always suffered from being stacked up without global order, and what is more of reintroducing into sexual matters truisms barely disguised in a falsely technical vocabulary. Here, the relentless pursuit of the unicity of the knot as manifest proof of the existence of a 'non-rapport' has come to grief on a stubborn fact: there is no way of obtaining such a unicity along the path of a flattening out. This, of course, does not prove the contrary, the inexistence of non-rapport, but leaves this latter without any other recourse than the enunciating that produced it.

'There is no sexual *rapport*' thus rejoins the other 'there is no' produced by Lacan throughout the years: 'there is no Other of the Other'; 'there is no metalanguage'. None of them can exhibit the object which would be valid as a proof for all bear witness to facts of internal limitations, which depend on the consistency of the predicated set and do not depend therefore on any *local* singularity that can be approached, be exhibited, of which one can 'make a case'. Each one of these statements nevertheless managed to subvert the operation of the universal and its particular by chipping away at the all thanks to which one can lay hold of any special one of its elements, which this all encompasses like a mother hen. In consequence, these same statements subvert the natural operation of the concept which calls for these objects, events, and individuals to gather together under her protective wings. Thus, they go against a whole literature in which the 'obsessional' disputes with the 'jealous person', who is differentiated or linked to the 'pervert', who happily takes the 'hysteric' as a partner, and so on. It opposes this psychopathological bestiary which displays its clinical entities, great consumers of 'cases' since these entities are fed by clinical vignettes as so many objects which 'fall' under them.

The non-rapport, to finish, has not found its object and remains an affirmation that must be referred to its enunciating – not just Jacques Lacan, in his idiosyncrasy, but also the totality of his teaching in which the precise conditions of this construction were forged. To export this enunciation to other ways of knowing, other practices, other styles, is not self-evident. The light that it projects on sexual difference has not made the starting ambiguity vary: yes, there are two sexes, quasi-independent (without 'rapport' with one another) and nevertheless held by a sort of no less imperative bond, in which these sexes may go as far as being interchanged: 'woman the colour of man', 'man the colour of woman'. The ungraspable and indubitable difference which separates and alienates them from one another does not assure any first identity of each one, any more than it dissolves it into a pure semblance. It is not on this that Lacan innovates; he maintains on this point the Freudian course in its fundamental equivocation.

On the contrary, on the logical construction of this difference, by writing the conceptual disequilibrium which at once distinguishes and joins them, he pushed very far the study of the formal network which allows two sexes as such to be posed. He even produced by that a sort of logical model of the sexual body by bringing back the manifest duality offered in procreation and generation to the symbolic tool by which every difference in the logical and conceptual order can be thought out. There is here a reversal of perspective – difficult to divine at first approach – similar to the one which makes us go from the idea of an ordered nature, deploying its necessities as it will, to that of an accidental evolution submitted to contingencies of every kind. Thus, one may marvel at the fact that the human being is sometimes so well in accord with his natural milieu, without further delaying on the fact that evolution has, in all its savagery, produced this suitability, sculpted among the range of possibles what had a chance of surviving, in order to offer to us this false pre-established harmony. In their fashion, the formulae of sexuation invite us to think of an immemorial time when the first logical articulations of a still-stumbling thought took their support on the strangeness of sexual distribution, and on the way that every social organisation of the human group has of responding to it, of channelling it, of warding off its equivocation by tying down its terms in canonical forms, which are never just right despite their efforts.

Notes

1 Rejoining thus, on a strictly formal plan, P. F. Strawson who, in his book *Individuals. An Essay in Descriptive Metaphysics*, put forward the idea of a 'non-relational bond' between subject and predicate.

2 See G. Le Gaufey, *L'Éviction de l'origine*, Paris, Epel, 1994, pp. 151–189. For the answer Lacan gives to Perelman about analogy, see pp. 172–177.

3 Another way of flattening-out of the Borromean knot into which each consistency sees its own circularity reduced to an infinite line in such a way that the set of over/under appears maintaining the property of the Borromean knotting: cut one . . .

INDEX

FSC
www.fsc.org
MIX
Papier | Fördert
gute Waldnutzung
FSC® C083411

Kolibri 360 GmbH
Ferdinand-Jühlke-Straße 7
99095 Erfurt, Deutschland
produktsicherheit@kolibri360.de